Keeping Faith in Faith-Based Organizations

Keeping Faith in Faith-Based Organizations
A Practical Theology of Salvation Army Health Ministry

Dean Pallant

WIPF & STOCK · Eugene, Oregon

KEEPING FAITH IN FAITH-BASED ORGANIZATIONS
A Practical Theology of Salvation Army Health Ministry

Copyright © 2012 Dean Pallant. All rights reserved. Except for brief quotations in critical publications or reviews, no part of this book may be reproduced in any manner without prior written permission from the publisher. Write: Permissions, Wipf and Stock Publishers, 199 W. 8th Ave., Suite 3, Eugene, OR 97401.

Wipf & Stock
An Imprint of Wipf and Stock Publishers
199 W. 8th Ave., Suite 3
Eugene, OR 97401

www.wipfandstock.com

ISBN 13: 978-1-61097-923-8

Manufactured in the U.S.A.

For my parents, David and Marion Pallant,
lifelong Salvationists and exemplars of living as 'healthy persons'

Contents

Foreword by Gary Gunderson ix
Preface by General Linda Bond xiii
Introduction xv

1 Identifying the Issues 1
2 Health for the Poorest People: The Contribution of the State and the Market 29
3 Health for the Poorest People beyond the State or the Market 52
4 Health for the Poorest People: Salvation Army Responses 88
5 A Soteriological Orientation for Health Ministry 125
6 Formulating Revised Forms of Practice 154

Bibliography and References 177
Index 187

Foreword

IF DEAN PALLANT'S BOOK was only useful for Salvation Army leaders, it would still be a bold work, drawing on carefully documented global investigation in that remarkable wide array of institutions that are the fruit of radical movement born in London in 1865, now planted in 124 nations. This is far more—and far more relevant—than an inside discussion intelligible only to those comfortable with the nuances of Salvationist discourse. Pallant's work is useful precisely because of its particularity, modeling for those in positions of influence of any faith-based organization a high order of reflection on practice using all the tools of mature reflection including theology inside and outside his own tradition, insights of social and medical scientists and a rich store of carefully observed work in the field. Finally, Pallant delivers the final stage of reflection—plainly written recommendations that can be acted on.

This book joins a still small but growing literature that many are surprised to find is still necessary in the twenty-first century, long past the time when social scientists expected religion and its institutions to be relevant for anyone other than historians to understand. But it turns out that religion matters because of its tools of theological reflection, its practices of institutional adaptation to hundreds of particular contexts, its capacity for moving coherently at global scale as an agent of change, its way of creating social spaces in which humans worship, think, care, and act as social bodies. Faith is of practical value when it is practiced and reflected on with integrity, as this book models.

Most would be satisfied with something less ambitious; perfectly happy with a handbook or catalog of "best practices" which are popular among those in a hurry to do good, raise money, or make problems go away. Pallant displays an inconvenient integrity that takes the whole religious phenomena seriously, including its theological and institutional roots. There is still a lot of hubris among the bio-medical elite, who believe too much in the efficacy of their pills and treatments designed to beat back death or disease. Pallant skips over the question of whether faith institutions can do useful things in the context of healthcare. In recent years it has been more common for governmental organizations at all levels to seek to plug in religious networks and institutions into their plans for responding to vast crises such as HIV/AIDS and a panoply of conditions ranging from suicide, hand-washing, immunizations, and obesity. It remains surprisingly common to hear of a researcher discovering that faith organizations are relevant to this or that community condition.

The Salvation Army has no need to argue for that with its many decades of living on the toughest streets in the world. The question Pallant wants us to struggle with is deceptively radical, shifting from a focus on disease to "healthy people." By the way, what is a healthy person? Who is best qualified to engage the question, much less build a field of practice on the answer? It may be possible to develop "best practices" to immunize populations without knowing a great deal about their rich complexity and diversity. Recent decades of public health experience suggest that even the most straightforward technical interventions fail because it turns out that people and their many-faceted social relationships are not made up of autonomous rational decision-makers responding to simply economic motivations. Religions knew about healthy people long before medical sciences developed the technical means to accelerate physical health at large scale. Pallant models the fact that religious language and patterns of thought are better for talking about healthy humans than biomedical technologists, not because faith institutions are better run, but because they begin with a more complex idea of what a human is, how we are together—and what we can become.

Pallant goes boldly where nobody really wants to go, toward congregations as agents of health, healing and, of course, salvation in its richest, most vital sense. Anyone who has ever tried to lead, or even attend a real congregation for more than a month or two would wish that science would have a pill to immunize us from having to enter into their radically unpredictable realities. Everything bad or frustrating about them is true. Libraries are filled with texts about the problematic nature of congregations. But if we did not already have hundreds of thousands of the peculiar social entities that are endemic to communities all over the globe, we would have to invent them to fulfill the promise of healthy people. The move toward congregations honors the confluence of science that needs relationships in order to work. Pallant sets out a list: "addictions, diabetes, disabilities, end-of-life care, eyes, HIV/AIDS, hypertension, infectious diseases, leprosy, maternal and child health, mental illness and nutrition." He will not let us have the instrumental power of faith-based organizations without paying attention to the *movement* that created them and continues to drive them into the future. Faith based movements are rooted in the places where faith is formed, nurtured and reimagined again and again—congregations.[1] Of course, congregations can be instrumentalized just as larger institutions are. But Pallant does not dumb them down into being tools of others' strategies; rather they are relevant because they are alive to and generative of faith experience in the social body.

Faith-based organizations are the last thing from static—they are themselves a form of life. And they are more; they derive from religious movements that are nurtured with the ancient constantly new social tools of worship, ritual, songs, poems, scripture, and a constant flow of wisdom literature. The *faith* part of *faith*-based organizations is constantly renewed, not safely left in the past. The faith part will be the future, or the movement will disappear as mist in the sun (an image common in the scripture of the Jewish people). Thus the reflection of the role of faith-based health organizations leads inexorably toward the congregation, the discipline of thought called "ecclesiology." What is the form and practice of faith operating at the base of faith? What science, techniques and practices relevant to health people should we hope to make normative there? Clarity about healthy people in relationship to each other and God lets us then imagine the more instrumental institutions we think of as higher: hospitals, clinics and the panoply of community health programs. Begin with an image of healthy people in healthy relationships; then imagine a movement of people carried forward on the Spirit of God to build the instruments God would hope for.

The Salvation Army has a particularly bold history on which to reflect—never fearing to be thought too odd or radical. Every faith is useful for imaging the future in a time when science offers us such extraordinarily useful tools. It is helpful to remember that every religion has been a movement bold in its place and times. Most can again move if they draw

---

1. I have written about the strengths of congregations that pertain to the health of communities in my book *Deeply Woven Roots* (Fortress Press, 1997).

on their own deep wells of hope and then engage the offerings of science and government as partners to be engaged from strength.

We are in a hurry these days to hammer our best practices together, scale them up to national and global programs. Pallant suggests there is nothing quite so useful as a movement with the capacity to reflect clearly on its practices and then move in radical faith as far as God illuminates.

May it be.

Gary Gunderson
Memphis, Tennessee, USA[2]

---

2. Rev Dr Gary Gunderson is Director for the Interfaith Health Program, Rollins School of Public Health, Emory University, Atlanta and Senior Vice President of Health and Welfare Ministries for Methodist Healthcare, USA.

Preface

THE SALVATION ARMY WILL soon celebrate its 150th anniversary. Serving in 124 countries, it enjoys the affirmation of those its serves and those it partners with, whether churches, NGOs or governments. While we are grateful, we must always guard against pride, inflexibility, or a relevance that is veiled compromise.

As long as we have Salvation Army officers like Major Dean Pallant, we need not fear. His loyalty does not muzzle him from an honest assessment of how and why and when we did not keep faith with our theological roots and gospel motivation. But he is a realistic optimist. His own personal faith, study, and experience qualify him as one who deserves to be heard. He envisions a "flexible, agile, ambitious Salvation Army movement, part of the wider Christian church, modeling a relevant, faithful, twenty-first century tension-building engagement in difficult situations resulting in an improvement in the health of the poorest people."

There is no sense of moaning about past failure or resting on our laurels or even presently committing to service that is mediocre at best. He speaks of a twenty-first century ministry of excellence and he calls The Salvation Army to a credible engagement with a view to making a difference. That difference will be the fruit of the work of effective, efficient, and resilient people who are clear on the *raison d'etre* of their movement. They understand that God in Jesus Christ offered a full salvation for the whole person, a relational salvation that effects change within a family, society, and even a nation. Transformation therefore need not be a pipe dream. Wholeness is the goal. When a Faith-Based Organization ministers out of a sound and practical theology, it is not only amazingly effective but it is blessed by God.

Though I have been challenged and encouraged by Dean's fresh approach, I would hasten to add that this book is not a word in season for The Salvation Army alone. It is timely for any Faith-Based Organization. The time has come for us to stand because of our faith in order to serve with compassion and grace.

General Linda Bond
International Leader of The Salvation Army, London

Introduction

I HAVE BEEN PRIVILEGED beyond measure in the past four years and this book is an attempt to share some of my many blessings with a wider audience. Two major events occurred in my life that changed my perspectives on many issues. First, my wife and I were appointed by The Salvation Army to review their health ministry around the world and develop an international vision and strategy. I have visited more than 40 countries in 4 years—what a privilege!

As we took up this appointment, I was studying for a doctorate in theology and ministry at King's College London. Under the guidance of a brilliant and supportive supervisor, Dr Luke Bretherton, I was able to combine my Salvation Army research task with my doctoral thesis. This book is the fruit of these two tasks.

My perspective on the health of the poorest people has changed in the past four years. I have visited numerous slums, many overcrowded cities and scores of isolated rural villages. From the hundreds, if not thousands, of people I have met on my travels, one child stands out in my memory. It was a hot, dusty afternoon in Kolkatta—the massive Indian city once called Calcutta. Unusually, I had a couple of hours free. I left the relative tranquility of my hostel and walked down a crowded, busy street to buy a bottle of water. Immediately, a very young boy, less than five years old, ran alongside me as I picked my way through the crowds. He shouted "Sweets, sweets!" I walked on. I had no sweets on me. As I bought my bottle of water from a street trader, I noticed he was also selling sweets. I bought a handful. As I returned down the pavement the boy appeared again. "Sweets?" he cried. He touched my hand and I was struck by the softness of the skin. I put my hands into my pocket and, like a wild animal, he lunged, grabbed them and ran off. I was stunned.

A child with such soft hands had already developed the skills and agility of a feral beast.

I should not have been surprised. The boy has probably lived on those tough streets since his birth. He developed the skills of survival. He had no choice. I never saw him again. Is he still alive?

He sticks in my memory and represents billions of people referenced in this academic work. I hope that in the midst of all the complex theory, detailed references and elaborate debate, the lives of individual people—such as the 'sweet' little boy in Kolkatta—will not be lost. These are real people, their plight is dire and the memory of that boy's soft skin coupled with cat-like reflexes motivates me when I feel weary.

This book unashamedly promotes a faith-inspired vision of a better world. Despite the billions of dollars spent on improving the health of the poorest people, the evidence of improvement is patchy and unsustainable in the face of economic turbulence. New approaches are desperately needed—the old approaches are too costly, overly bureaucratic and ineffective. The resources of faith must be brought to the task. This book describes a way this can happen and uses current Salvation Army situations to show how.

I hope readers find it has application well beyond The Salvation Army. This is a tradition-specific piece of practical theology. It has to be. That was my task. However, the methodology and literature referenced in this book have application for other faith-based groups—hence the title, *Keeping Faith In Faith-Based Organizations*. The task is too big for The Salvation Army alone. All people of faith are needed, as are their faith resources.

I acknowledge all the encouragement, insights, and advice from many friends, colleagues and family in the writing of this book. First, I acknowledge my friend, fellow Salvationist, and practical theologian Dr Helen Cameron. Helen has been a consistent encouragement and I could not have completed this book—and the doctorate in theology resourcing my research—without Helen's mentorship. Dr Brian Brock and Dr Stephen Plant examined my doctoral thesis. I acknowledge with sincere thanks their in-depth analysis and recommendations for improvement. I have included a number of their insights in this book.

Many unnamed but perceptive people around the world helped me appreciate the complexity and potential of Salvation Army health ministry. I am deeply grateful for each one. Two Salvation Army officers require special acknowledgement for their long-term contribution to my personal development. Commissioner (Dr) Paul du Plessis and Commissioner John Swinfen have shared many significant conversations with me over a period of more than 20 years. These two wise, gifted, and experienced Salvation Army leaders have given lifetimes of service in developing world countries. I am particularly grateful they were willing to comment on a draft of this book. I will continue to be grateful for their friendship and wisdom.

I acknowledge, with sincere thanks, the significant support provided by The Salvation Army for my doctoral studies and the completion of this book. I also thank my aunt, Alison Brown, a professional indexer, for her gift of this book's index.

Finally, my wife Eirwen, and children, Laurence and Rachel, deserve special acknowledgment for their patience, support, and love throughout the hectic, crazy past few years. I love you all very much.

Dean Pallant
London, New Year's Day, 2012

1

Identifying the Issues

FAITH-BASED ORGANIZATIONS (FBOs) ARE receiving attention in the global quest for better health for the world's poorest people. Governments are increasingly partnering with FBOs to achieve domestic and foreign policy objectives. There is appreciation of the high levels of trust many of the poorest people have in FBOs—with 82 percent preferring FBOs to non-faith groups in a recent survey in sub-Saharan Africa.[1] The World Bank published research noting higher quality of service and lower prices from FBO health providers in Uganda.[2] The Bill and Melinda Gates Foundation funded research into the reach and effectiveness of FBOs, noting that between 30 and 70 percent of health institutions in Africa are "in the hands of religious entities."[3] This assessment of the impact of FBOs is widely accepted and quoted.[4] A number of academic disciplines are currently engaging with the complex task of defining, mapping, and evaluating the contribution of FBOs to global health.[5] Partnerships with faith-based groups are increasing but there is concern that "enthusiasm for partnership has run ahead of the knowledge of the nature, scope,

---

1. DFID, "Religion 'Good for Development.'"
2. Reinikka and Svensson, "Working for God?," 1.
3. Olivier et al., "Working in a Bounded Field of Unknowing," 33.
4. World Health Organization, "Building from Common Foundations," 9. UNAIDS, "Partnership with Faith Based Organizations," 8.
5. Olivier, "In Search of Common Ground," 80.

and scale of religious entities and religious response, not to mention their unique characteristics that may demand a specific strategy."[6]

The definition and use of the term "Faith-Based Organization" is contested and controversial. The terms "Religious Entities" and "Religious Assets" have been proposed as alternatives.[7] However, this book uses FBO given the priority this descriptor gives to matters of *faith*. Included within my definition of FBO is every group or organization that claims to operate from a faith-base beyond the worshipping community. Therefore, local congregations are not included within my definition of FBOs but I include a myriad of organizations who claim a faith-base including schools, hospitals, clinics, grassroots community development groups, advocacy organizations, national coordinating bodies, multi-national development agencies, etc. My priority is not to assess organizational capacity but, rather, the contribution of *faith*.[8]

Unlike much of the current research into FBOs working in the developing world, this book is not primarily seeking to determine how to improve the efficiency or effectiveness of the FBOs in terms of achieving global health objectives. I do not accept that FBOs should adopt objectives and policies set by politicians and government officials; nor simply determine program priorities according to the funding criteria of the world's wealthiest people; nor embrace the business models of large commercial health providers. Although the actions of state and market inevitably impact FBOs, the direction and character of a Faith-Based Organization should by definition, be determined by matters of faith. Therefore, the theology of a Faith-Based Organization should be the primary influence on an FBO. If its *faith* does not drive an FBO, whose *faith* does?

---

6. Ibid., 84.

7. Ibid., 89.

8. The complexity of defining FBOs is highlighted in the case of The Salvation Army, who defines itself officially in *The 2010 Salvation Army Year Book* as "an international movement, an evangelical part of the universal Christian Church" with a mission to "preach the gospel of Jesus Christ and meet human needs in his name without discrimination" (The Salvation Army, 2009, iii). However, as will be discussed later, there is a tendency towards fragmentation between the congregation who "preach" and the social services who "meet human needs."

THE CONTEXT: THE EXPERIENCE OF THE SALVATION ARMY

In October 2007, my wife and I were appointed International Health Services Coordinators for The Salvation Army. I have been a Salvation Army officer since my ordination and commissioning in 1993. My wife, Eirwen—a medical doctor and Salvation Army officer—and I received the appointment to International Headquarters tasked with developing an international vision and strategy for Salvation Army health ministry. It is not unusual in The Salvation Army for husband and wife to work together although we are the first couple to jointly hold this appointment.

The Salvation Army is a denomination of the Christian church working in more than 120 countries with many health programs. Globally this includes 29 general hospitals, 25 maternity hospitals, 19 other specialist hospitals, 56 specialist clinics, 135 health centers, 64 mobile clinics, and more than 15,000 local congregations (usually called corps) almost all of whom have a community service program.[9]

Unlike most Christian denominations, The Salvation Army has a global governance structure with every unit and program ultimately accountable to one person—the General. During initial briefings, senior Salvation Army leaders expressed concern that many Salvation Army hospitals and clinics in economically developing countries were declining in their quality of service and were not financially sustainable. There was some internal disagreement on the way forward. For a number of years priority had been given to community-based rather than hospital-based health ministry. Community-based health care was more fundable, less risky, and perceived to be more effective and sustainable. In the past 25 years, The Salvation Army withdrew from almost all hospital-based health care in economically developed countries. Leaders responsible for the closures justified their actions on the grounds of increasing cost, the threat of lawsuits, and conflict with state grant makers and regulators over human life ethics. A number of influential western voices were recommending the closure of all Salvation Army hospitals around the world.

Salvationists in developing countries overwhelmingly disagreed with closure proposals. The arguments for improving institutional-based health ministry were justified on more than mere emotional attachment to institutions with a long and glorious past—although that driver should not be minimized. Salvationists expressed a desire to continue

---

9. The Salvation Army, *The Salvation Army Year Book 2010*, 30.

to serve poor and marginalized people through institutional, corps, and community-based health ministry by offering a continuous chain of care from home to hospital and back. Institutional-based health ministry was justified on the basis that hospitals and clinics give The Salvation Army credibility and provide a valuable space in the public square for ministry—particularly in Christian-minority settings where people of other faiths sometimes view Salvation Army corps and community-based initiatives with suspicion. An Indonesian Salvation Army officer, Major Yusak Tampai, explained this argument during my visit to Indonesia in January 2008. His presentation was a key moment in challenging my thinking on the role of hospitals and clinics in 21st-century health ministry.

In addition to concerns about the future of health institutions, several leaders in economically "developed" and "developing" contexts expressed unease at the increasing influence of secularist development thinking in Salvation Army health and development programs. Some leaders felt the communities' capacity to solve their problems was being overestimated while health and development practitioners were sidelining theological resources.

The Salvation Army is not the only FBO facing this challenge. Stephen Plant identifies similar trends in other Christian agencies and suggests some are replacing Christian eschatology with a "secular eschatology" derived from non-religious, non-governmental organizations.[10] Secular eschatology promotes hope, without any requirement for God and a "belief in human progress" with trust invested in concepts such as the capacity of science, the capacity of humanity, and human rights to secure a better world.

Plant notes how "the seed of Christian hope of salvation grew into the bush of a belief in human progress"[11] and suggests that, despite significant differences, it is possible to find commonality between secular development (defined as belief in progress) with the Christian eschatological hope. Plant does not hide the tensions between secular belief in progress and Christian development work and argues Christians need to tread a careful path between two heresies: "On the one hand, Christians must resist those who advocate the eschewal of all political questions (such as development) as belonging to a fallen material world; on the other, they

10. Plant, "Freedom as Development: Christian Mission and the Definition of Human Well-Being," 1.
11. Idem., "International Development and Belief in Progress," 849.

must resist the notion that human beings may work out their own salvation on earth. Christians, that is, have a proper penultimate interest in life before death, but their ultimate peace and fulfillment as human beings lies in the love of God."[12]

In the framing of community health and development initiatives, Plant notes that FBOs often promote the notion that human beings can work out their own salvation compounded by a reticence to refer to a "faith" dimension for fear of accusations of evangelism. Plant argues: "The rich resources of Christian theology fail to have much if any discernible bearing upon the policies and practices of church-based development agencies. Christian theology has available to it a palate of rich color; but many Christian development practitioners, in making social justice their only theological rationale, seem content to paint in monochrome."[13]

Stanley Hauerwas offers a trenchant critique of Christian motive and practice in his assessment of the reasons for the growing popularity of social justice among western Christians. He argues that the current emphasis "springs not so much from an effort to locate the Christian contribution to wider society as it does from Christian's attempts to find a way to be societal actors without that action being colored by Christian presuppositions."[14]

Paul Gifford, in a recent ethnography of contemporary African Christianity, provides detailed analysis of the extent to which the Kenyan Church is engaged in the "development business" but notes very few FBOs in Kenya "seem interested in even asking whether there is any specifically Christian way of or contribution to development."[15] Gifford, who claims not to have a theological or denominational interest in his study, reaches a disturbing conclusion: "[The] increasing identification of mainline Christianity with Western development aid is something whose significance needs to be acknowledged. As Africa has become increasingly marginalized, excluded from globalizing movements and processes, these aid flows and what they involve have become increasingly significant for, even constitutive of, parts of mainline Christianity. This is the sense in which one can talk of secularization in Africa. It is

---

12. Ibid., 853.
13. Idem., "Does Faith Matter in Development?," 3.
14. Hauerwas, *After Christendom?*, 58.
15. Gifford, *Christianity, Politics and Public Life in Kenya*, 49.

not that Africans are notably becoming secularized, but much of mainline Christianity effectively is."[16]

As field reflections in this book will show, similar challenges confront The Salvation Army around the world. In 2004, Brian Howe critiqued The Salvation Army in Australia noting that if it were a company The Salvation Army would easily be one of Australia's top 200. Howe claims that despite its incredible success, The Salvation Army in Australia is on a "knife-edge" arguing that corporate and financial success has become the basis for too many decisions. Howe writes: "This is not to say The Salvation Army or other church-based welfare agencies do not provide effectively and efficiently important social welfare services, it is rather the freedom of the church to be the church which is threatened by its accommodation to the demands of a corporatist or a market-related culture. What room is left for the church to represent an alternative voice? Where is the necessary tension between church and society?"[17]

Howe poses a challenging question: To what extent has the twenty-first century Salvation Army accommodated corporate or political agendas? This book seeks to provide resources to resist such accommodation.

I have observed reluctance among many FBO practitioners to articulate the difference that faith makes in their practice. During the writing of this book, I have discussed this issue with employees from several FBOs. Many are wary of theology and the church taking a central role in policy and practice. "Faith" is left as a loose, undefined label rather than imbued with richness from theological resources such as the Bible and Church tradition coupled with the habits and practices of people enabled by the power of the Holy Spirit.

Many FBO practitioners promote the instrumental capacity of the church to reach vulnerable people but perceive church leaders and theology as barriers to their priorities of effective and efficient initiatives to improve the health of poor people.[18] Most FBOs have accepted partnerships with the global public health establishment who appear, in effect, to view faith-based groups (including congregations and

---

16. Ibid., 50.

17. Howe, "Politics and Faith: Living in Truth," 44.

18. Viewing the church as one of a number of community groups rather than the prime partner for FBO health work was the World Vision strategy as explained to me at the 2008 International AIDS Conference in Mexico City by one of their leading AIDS program managers in Africa.

denominational infrastructure) as simply an effective distribution network for secular initiatives.

FBOs appear to prioritize their value as *organization* above their contribution as a repository of *faith*. Even Tearfund—one of the most faith-based of FBOs[19]—uses instrumental terms to describe the local church's contribution to the fight against HIV/AIDS. The following definition of the church comes from a Tearfund report seeking to share "examples of good practice" and "facilitate greater understanding of the significant contribution of the church in response to HIV."[20]

> The Christian church is an existing and sustainable grassroots network with unparalleled reach and authority in many local communities. Working with the local church provides a unique opportunity to mobilize thousands of volunteers and scale up responses to HIV. The local church has the potential to effectively disseminate information, influence attitudes, and values, advocate with and on behalf of the vulnerable and reach marginalized populations."[21]

The document contains scant reference to God, the resources of the faith tradition or the habits and practices of people of faith that form the "attitudes and values" or sustain the church's "unparalleled reach and authority."[22] However, this book will show a purely instrumental description of the contribution of the church is theologically deficient.

FBOs appear to lack the resources to engage in meaningful dialogue in an inter-disciplinary conversation with public health. Reflecting on more than five years of such conversations in the African Religious Health Assets Programme (ARHAP), Olivier writes: "In collaborative communication, PH (Public Health) discourse appears to be more powerful than that of RS (Religious Studies) not only because of its links to scientific institutions of power, but also because of its narrative authoritative style. Hermeneutics, interpretation, and reflection does not fare well when it comes into competition with a discourse of certain authority."[23]

---

19. Tearfund's website states they are "passionate about living out God's kingdom values," promotes classical evangelical Christian doctrinal statements and prioritizes working with local churches as partners (www.tearfund.org).
20. Tearfund, "Transforming Lives: Church-Based Responses to HIV," 1.
21. Ibid., 28.
22. Ibid., 1.
23. Olivier, "In Search of Common Ground," 133.

Between October 2007 and December 2011, I travelled extensively to Salvation Army health programs visiting all five continents and spending many hours with hundreds of people discussing the current state and future hopes for faith-based health ministry. I visited programs in India, Bolivia, Zambia, Zimbabwe and Indonesia (a number of visits to these countries), Papua New Guinea, Fiji, Tonga, The Philippines, Bangladesh, Sri Lanka, Democratic Republic of Congo, South Africa, Ghana, Kenya (twice), Rwanda, Argentina, Brazil, Paraguay, Mexico, Haiti (twice), Sweden, Norway, New Zealand, and USA. I also visited Canada, Australia, Netherlands, Switzerland, UK, and Hong Kong for discussions with senior leaders overseeing health and social ministry. In addition to these field visits, insights were gained at the Global Health Conference in Washington DC in May 2008, the International World AIDS Conference in Mexico City in August 2008 and meetings between Non Government Organizations (NGOs) and Faith-Based Organizations (FBOs) at the World Health Organization (WHO) in Geneva in October 2008 and November 2009. In particular, I acknowledge valuable learning at the Christian Connections for International Health Conference (CCIH) in Washington DC in May 2008 and May 2010 and the Africa Religious Health Assets Programme (ARHAP) Colloquium held in Cape Town, South Africa in July 2009.

During all these experiences I sought to understand, explore, and investigate the myriad of challenges facing FBOs seeking to improve the health of the poorest people in the developing world and the competing visions of the best way forward being proposed by governments, for-profit organizations, non-governmental groups as well as faith and non-faith community-based groups. The temptation to settle for "thin" one-dimensional understandings of health was resisted, as this would fail to do justice to the complexity confronting the poorest people's quest for better health. At every opportunity, I noted down facts, impressions, and reflections and at the end of each day dictated my reflections that were later typed up. These notes do not constitute primary data for the book but they assisted, enriched, and informed my understanding of the factors affecting The Salvation Army's ability to conduct faithful health ministry in the twenty-first century. All of this contributed to the process of reflective practice, with the results recorded in this book.

RESEARCH METHOD: A PRACTICAL THEOLOGICAL REFLECTION

In recent years there has been an increasing appreciation of the value of reflection in professional practice as against a "technical rationalist" approach.[24] The reflective practitioner approach has been adopted in a wide range of disciplines including medicine, engineering, architecture, education, social work, and practical theology. Schön identified an important distinction between reflection-in-action (where the practitioner draws on internalized theory to make an in-the-moment decision) and reflection-on-action, which enables a retrospective review leading to an evaluation of action and revised practice.[25]

Given the priority of faith in this book, I use a methodology grounded within the discipline of practical theology for a reflection-on-action. Practical theology is a diverse and developing field.[26] It recognizes the importance of the complex dynamics of the contemporary human experience and seeks a more faithful *performance* of the gospel[27] rather than confining theology to an historic engagement with sacred texts and traditions.

There are a number of ways of doing theology to take account of the experience of the past (the texts and traditions) and the experience of the present (the context in which Christians of a concrete time and place find themselves).[28] Stephen Bevans, in seeking a global perspective for theology, identifies at least six different models ranging from an Anthropological Model that prioritizes the preservation of cultural identity by a person of Christian faith to a Translation Model whose primary concern is the preservation of Christian identity while taking context seriously.[29] I sought a methodology that valued human experience as a place where the gospel is "grounded, embodied, interpreted, and lived out."[30] Bevans identifies this as the Praxis Model—a means of not simply interpreting the world, but changing it. Scripture and Tradition are understood not merely as

---

24. Schon, *The Reflective Practitioner*, 22ff.
25. Thompson, *SCM Studyguide to Theological Reflection*, 22.
26. Pattison and Woodward, "Introduction to Pastoral and Practical Theology," 16.
27. Swinton and Mowat, *Practical Theology and Qualitative Research*, 4.
28. Bevans, *An Introduction to Theology in Global Perspectives*, 166.
29. Ibid., 174.
30. Swinton and Mowat, *Practical Theology and Qualitative Research*, 5.

"vehicles of revelation" but rather "models of action" that invite believers to "join God in God's liberating and saving activity within the weave of human and cosmic history."[31] The Praxis Model offers an appropriate methodology to engage in critical theological reflection on the practices of health ministry in The Salvation Army by giving opportunity for theological resources to engage with the practice of health services to ensure and enable "more faithful participation in God's work of redemption in, to, and for the world."[32]

The Praxis Model seeks to critically interpret situations and practices.[33] This requires taking an issue that at first glance may appear to be uncomplicated but after a process of critical reflection at various levels is complex and polyvalent.[34] The issues surrounding the health of the poorest people are certainly complex and polyvalent. To adequately interpret the situation and, hopefully, enable more faithful practice, this book engages with a number of other academic disciplines in particular development studies, public health, and political theology. The research base for the book is, therefore, a critical engagement with a variety of literature, informed by personal reflection, and driven by a desire to ensure and enable Salvation Army health ministry's faithful participation in God's redemptive practices in, to, and for the world.

The choice of a multidisciplinary approach might be criticized for lacking depth in a particular academic discipline. However due to the reality and complexity of international Salvation Army health ministry it was essential to seek complexity of breadth by engaging with a number of academic disciplines in preference to complexity in depth which would focus on one academic specialty.

To structure the book, Swinton and Mowat's four-stage model of practical theological reflection[35] is used. The four stages are:

- *Stage One* (Current praxis) identifies a situation that requires reflection and critical challenge.
- *Stage Two* (Cultural/contextual analysis) begins the process of

---

31. Bevans, *An Introduction to Theology in Global Perspectives*, 178.

32. Swinton and Mowat, *Practical Theology and Qualitative Research*, 6.

33. For an overview of the development and theological foundations of the Praxis Model see Graham, Walton, and Ward, *Theological Reflection: Methods*, 170–99.

34. Swinton and Mowat, *Practical Theology and Qualitative Research*, 13.

35. Ibid., 95.

entering into dialogue with a range of sources of knowledge to develop a deeper understanding of the situation.

- *Stage Three* (Theological Reflection) allow for a critical reflection on the practices of church and world in the light of Scripture and tradition. The search is for "authentic revelation in a spirit of critical faithfulness and chastened optimism."[36]

- *Stage Four* (Formulating revised practice) attempts to draw together the cultural/contextual analysis with theological reflections in a conversation, producing new forms of more faithful practice.

There is considerable back and forth between the stages in the process of describing, analyzing, theologically reflecting, and formulating proposals for revised practice. The research did not follow a linear progression from issue to social scientific analysis and then to theology. Three of the six chapters of this book focus on the cultural/contextual analysis stage.

However, this does not mean theological reflection is absent until Chapter 5. The earlier chapters contain many insights from theology. In adopting this approach, I am attentive to the possibility of God's agency in the work of describing and analyzing the culture and context within which Salvation Army health ministry operates. After Bretherton, I reject any confinement of theology to "the analysis of data generated by supposedly neutral social scientific methods."[37]

Writing this book while holding a position of responsibility within The Salvation Army raised some methodological issues. Although my "insider" position offered access to the inner processes and practice of Salvation Army health ministry with information inaccessible to an external researcher, I needed to be alert to the risks and potential pitfalls of bias.[38] However, by seeking an insider-outsider perspective I was able to gain a fuller understanding of the complex nuances and challenges facing Salvation Army health ministry. The distinction between "insiders" and "outsiders" is rarely clear-cut and the role of "insiders" is particularly

---

36. Ibid., 96.
37. Bretherton, *Christianity and Contemporary Politics*, 30.
38. Denscombe, *The Good Research Guide*, 63.

constructive in researching faith-based groups.[39] Aware of issues of bias, my analysis was triangulated using a multidisciplinary literature review.

The "insider" position enabled me to use a number of tools to reflect on the issues that were raised. I dictated initial reflections at the end of each day during the intensive research phase between October 2007 and December 2009. After each visit a report, including a summary of the information gathered, key conclusions, and recommendations for revised practice, was shared with International Salvation Army leaders in London and in the locations visited. On a number of occasions, leaders wrote back with comments and provided more information to improve my analysis. I took a camera on each visit and have taken thousands of pictures in the past three years. I shared some pictures on a social networking site and received a number of reactions from people to the images.[40] All of this information was helpful in enriching my understanding of the context of Salvation Army practice. I co-facilitated a number of workshops[41] that gave me the opportunity to reflect back to a significant number of key Salvation Army practitioners my initial conclusions. In the light of their input, I revised my thinking. I could have adopted a more qualitative analysis of data but I decided a better approach was to use a reflective process of description, analysis and reflection to answer the task set by the leaders of The Salvation Army—how can a theologically faithful future for health ministry be defined and achieved?

INTRODUCING THE ISSUE: THE HEALTH OF THE POOREST PEOPLE

Overall, the world's population is healthier, wealthier, and lives longer today than 30 years ago. *The World Health Report 2008* notes that if children were still dying at 1978 rates, there would have been 16.2 million deaths globally in 2006. In fact, there were "only" 9.5 million child deaths. The improvement is attributed by the World Health Organization (WHO) to the provision of essential drugs and significant improvements in access to clean water, sanitation, and antenatal care. There has also been a 35 percent growth in the world's health expenditure

---

39. Stringer, "Introduction: Theorizing Faith," 16.

40. www.facebook.com/pallant.

41. Hong Kong (November 2008); Coonoor, India (May 2009); Geelong, Australia (October 2009); Ascension, Paraguay (November 2009); Kakamega, Kenya (May 2010).

between 2000 and 2005, increased knowledge and understanding of health on the back of the technological revolution and much better international partnerships for health as exemplified by the commitment in the Millennium Development Goals (MDGs) to eliminate poverty.[42] The optimistic conclusion to be drawn from this evidence could be that, given the right resources and conditions, it is possible to improve the health of the poorest people.

However, the WHO identifies other less optimistic trends. The substantial progress in health has been deeply unequal with a considerable number of countries lagging behind the progress achieved by others—some countries are even losing ground. Furthermore, there is much research—not available 30 years ago—of considerable and often growing health inequalities within countries. In Nairobi, for example, the under-five mortality rate is below 15 per 1,000 in high-income areas. In a slum in the same city, the rate is 254 per 1,000.[43] Despite billions of dollars in aid given each year, preventable diseases such as malaria and diarrhea result in almost 11 million deaths per year in poor countries.[44] Comparisons between the United Kingdom and Sub-Saharan Africa are shocking: "Child deaths under 5: in Sub-Saharan Africa 179 in 1000; in UK 6 in 1000. Life expectancy for a woman: in Sub-Saharan Africa 46; in UK 78. Annual health expenditure per person: in Sub-Saharan Africa US$ 36; in UK US$ 2,231."[45]

The prime cause of death for women in poor countries is pregnancy and childbirth—resulting in the death of more than 500,000 women every year. These health issues continue to disproportionately afflict people in the poorest countries (countries with per capita income below US$825 in 2006), which account for the majority (56 percent) of the global disease burden.[46] In fact, it is incorrect to talk about one homogeneous disease burden. There are three disease burdens simultaneously affecting much of the developing world—the continuing burden of communicable diseases,

---

42. World Health Organization, "The World Health Report 2008," xii ff.
43. Ibid., 7.
44. Schiber et al., "Financing Global Health: Mission Unaccomplished," 921.
45. Crisp, "Global Health Partnerships," 208.
46. Schiber et al., "Financing Global Health: Mission Unaccomplished," 921.

the increasing burden of chronic diseases, and increasing demand for both primary and tertiary levels of health care services.[47]

Analysis by health economists reveals most public health spending going to the non-poor with much of it failing to reach frontline service providers. When money does reach the frontline, providers have few incentives to deliver services effectively.[48] The preference for disease specific funding applied through a vertical funding stream (for example, AIDS, TB or Malaria) has highlighted the weakness of health systems in many developing countries. The World Health Organization argues: "Global and, increasingly, national policy formulation processes have focused on single issues, with various constituencies competing for scarce resources, while scant attention is given to the underlying constraints that hold up health systems development in national contexts. Rather than improving their response capacity and anticipating new challenges, health systems seem to be drifting from one short-term priority to another, increasingly fragmented, and without a clear sense of direction."[49]

Failing health systems affects the health of the poorest people in different ways. Firstly, health systems—where a command-and-control approach to disease control focused on short-term results—tend to fragment service delivery.[50] For example, significant concerns are surfacing that massive imbalances have been caused by HIV/AIDS funding. Although some argue the overall increase in global health aid in the period 1992–2005 has mitigated this to some extent,[51] it is difficult to deny the substantial disruption caused to other health and social services by the unprecedented resources available for AIDS.[52] Secondly, there is a disproportionate focus on specialist, tertiary care, often referred to as "hospital-centrism" which impacts the health of the poorest people.[53] There is significant resistance across the world to shifting resources away from hospitals. As a group of informed researchers wryly note: "The

47. Islam and Zaffar Tahir, "Health Sector Reform in South Asia," 151.

48. Center for Global Development, "Does the IMF Constrain Health Spending in Poor Countries?," 4.

49. World Health Organization, "The World Health Report 2008," xiii.

50. Ibid.

51. Shiffman, "Has Donor Prioritization of HIV/AIDS Displaced Aid for Other Health Issues?," 95.

52. Easterly, *The White Man's Burden*, 224.

53. World Health Organization, "The World Health Report 2008," 13.

problems of hospitals [in Africa] will be resolved with great difficulty, a factor which must contribute to an explanation of the low level of interest in the subject."[54]

Thirdly, the failure of health systems where a hands-off or laissez-faire approach to governance has allowed unregulated commercialization of health to flourish is seriously impacting the health of the poorest people.[55] These trends should not be simplistically attributed to the effects of state policy. There is undoubtedly also significant influence from the market, the local community and external donors in shaping the health systems—albeit perhaps unintentionally—to the detriment of the poorest people. The WHO argues these trends undermine efforts to build a comprehensive and balanced health program and will need to be addressed if the health of the poorest is to be improved. The fear is that in a number of countries, "the resulting inequitable access, impoverishing costs, and erosion of trust in health care constitute a threat to social stability."[56]

The health statistics for the poorest people are a major cause for concern for FBOs, like The Salvation Army, who prioritize the health needs of poor and marginalized people.[57] People of faith and their organizations have a long history of partnering with the state to improve the health of the poorest people. However, the current shape of state-faith relations needs careful consideration. Bretherton provides an analysis of the broader context of the turn to civil society in North America and Western Europe[58] and similar trends can be noted in western governmental policy in global health initiatives.

FBOs are perceived to be a "useful" asset for the cause of global health because, firstly, people of faith have access to many of the most inaccessible communities and are seen as a means for reducing inequitable access. Second, FBOs claim to operate a more effective and efficient service. Given the weight of religious teaching encouraging followers to

---

54. Hanson et al., "Towards Improving Hospital Performance in Uganda and Zambia," 75.

55. World Health Organization, "The World Health Report 2008," xiii.

56. Ibid.,

57. The international vision statement for Salvation Army health ministry issued in October 2008 states: "The Salvation Army seeks to be a significant participant in faith-based, integrated, quality primary health care as close to the family as possible giving priority to poor and marginalized members of society."

58. Bretherton, *Christianity and Contemporary Politics*, 32–37.

serve others it would be unsurprising if faith-groups could not tap into reservoirs of "social capital."[59] This should give FBOs a quantifiable advantage in a cost-benefit analysis as against a commercial or state provider.[60] Third, declining levels of trust in state and market sector health services by the poorest people,[61] present FBOs with an opportunity to offer a distinctive health ministry and, in so doing, improve the health of the poorest people who are a cause of significant public health concern and interest.[62]

The turn towards FBOs has been supported by voices within the global health establishment critiquing the priority given to rational individualism in western medicine and the influence of epidemiological and biomedical frameworks. This rational individualism is viewed by public health academics to be "of limited assistance in understanding the internal dynamics of health systems . . . The core behavioral assumption of traditional economic analysis, that human behavior is primarily rational and calculative, is flawed."[63] The discipline of public health is focusing on the importance of trust as "a relational notion between people. The motivational basis for trust is presented as including some combination of strong personal bonds and the belief that it enhances our own interests."[64] While most faith-based groups would promote a motivation higher than merely self-interest, the need to rebuild trust levels in wider society—as well as improve the access and affordability of health provision—fits well with the values motivating FBOs.

Over the years, faith-based practitioners and organizations have made significant contributions in focusing public health strategy on Primary Health Care (PHC). In September 1978, the nations of the world signed a joint declaration at Alma-Ata pledging to improve health for the poorest people through PHC defined as "essential health care based on practical, scientifically sound, and socially acceptable methods and

---

59. Putnam, *Bowling Alone*, 15–47.

60. This book is not attempting to research this claim but it is worth noting USA-based studies reporting conflicting evidence Kennedy, "Privatization and Prayer," 5–19.

61. Birungi, "Injections and Self-Help," 1455–62., Davies, "Falling Public Trust in Health Services," 193–94. Segall, "From Cooperation to Competition in National Health Systems-and Back?," 61–79.

62. Gilson, "Trust and the Development of Health Care as a Social Institution," 1456.

63. Ibid., 1453.

64. Ibid., 1456.

technology made universally accessible to individuals and families in the community through their full participation and at a cost the community and country can afford to maintain at every stage of their development in the spirit of self-reliance and self-determination."[65]

There was significant influence from people of faith in the development of the Alma-Ata declaration.[66] However, almost as soon as the Alma-Ata Conference was over, PHC was under attack. The central principle of enabling communities in developing countries to have responsibility for planning and implementing their own healthcare services was viewed as idealistic and costly. Selective Primary Health Care (SPHC) was a compromise solution focusing on reducing the rate of mortality of children through activities such as growth monitoring, oral rehydration solutions, breastfeeding and immunization. However, this took decision-making power and control away from the grassroots level and gave it to "foreign consultants with technical expertise in these specific areas."[67]

There were other reasons why PHC did not achieve the target of "Health For All by the Year 2000." Many "ordinary" people perceived PHC to be a cheap form of healthcare and, wherever possible, bypassed the under equipped and understaffed clinic to attend hospital. Civil war, natural disasters and, more recently, HIV affected the ability of PHC to maintain services. Governments perceived PHC as a way to reduce health expenditure but lacked the will to shift resources from expensive urban-based hospitals. Serious levels of corruption and poor governance resulted in donors being very wary of funding comprehensive, broad-based programs. Vertical, definable, time-limited programs that could be changed every few years suited both donor agencies and governments.[68]

In 2008, the WHO launched a revised PHC approach accepting it is still the best way to improve the health of the poorest people because PHC recognizes the importance of the social value of health systems.[69] The WHO *World Health Report 2008* identifies four interlocking sets of PHC reforms. Firstly, achieve universal access and social protection, so as to improve health equity. Secondly, re-organize service delivery around

65. World Health Organization, "Declaration of Alma-Ata International Conference," 2.
66. Taylor-Ide and Taylor, *Just and Lasting Change*, 5.
67. Hall and Taylor, "Health for All Beyond 2000," 18.
68. Ibid., 18–19.
69. World Health Organization, "The World Health Report 2008," 100.

people's needs and expectations. Thirdly, remodel leadership for health around more effective government securing healthier communities through better public policies.[70] The fourth set of reforms center on the importance of the active participation of key stakeholders—and includes FBOs. The WHO has indicated this opens up an opportunity for FBO participation but the nature and terms of participation are unclear. Recent events suggest the WHO integrated primary health care initiative appears to have been sidelined by the latest popularist "single issue"—maternal and child health—which was made the priority by world leaders at the UN Heads of Government summit in New York in September 2010.[71] However, if all the health issues affecting the poorest women and children are responded to with an integrated PHC approach, this may be a positive development.

To summarize: this section has identified a situation requiring reflection and critical challenge—the health of the world's poorest people. A number of issues that reduce the opportunity for poor people to enjoy health have been noted: fragmented disease specific interventions; high-cost of health services driven up by specialist and commercial interests; inaccessible populations; ineffective and inefficient providers; a decline in trust in health providers. There is a desire from many people to do something about this. This book will develop a faith-based response to this dire situation enabling FBOs to engage with clarity and confidence in this critically important issue.

WHAT IS THE QUESTION—IDENTITY, LOCATION, OR ORIENTATION?

Research should be initiated when there is a "living contradiction"; feeling dissonance that "we are not acting in accordance with our values and beliefs."[72] During visits to a number of Salvation Army health programs around the world, I sensed such a living contradiction. It appeared that many Salvation Army programs were influenced by what Alistair MacIntyre, in his analysis of contemporary moral debate, called "a set of incoherent, fragmented survivals from moral knowledge, and

---

70. Ibid., 148.
71. United Nations, "The Global Strategy for Women's and Children's Health," 1–20.
72. McNiff et al., *You and Your Action Research Project*, 59.

tradition."⁷³ Against an incoherent, fragmented worldview, The Salvation Army requires a common, clearly articulated, and sustainable health ministry applicable in every context around the world.

Given the increased attention to questions of space in recent theological literature,⁷⁴ my initial intention was to seek a "faithful location" for Salvation Army health ministry. I hoped that by establishing a universal, faithful occupation of space and location, The Salvation Army would be better able to sustain faithful relationships with state, market, communities, NGOs, and other FBOs. Space is "produced by people performing operations on places, using things in different ways for different ends."⁷⁵ Different spaces are produced according to "the stories that organize the play of changing relationships."⁷⁶ As Augustine conceived, the Church inhabits an alternate space that is in tension with the citizenship of the world.⁷⁷ William Cavanaugh has developed a contemporary treatment of Augustine's argument. He argues the Church is not in competition with the world because the world forfeited any claim to be truly public by its refusal to give God his due.⁷⁸

However, as I began to work with the concept of space, its geographical overtones presented a rigidity that was restrictive. The concept tended towards a sense of arriving at the destination, with an overemphasis on defending space. My intention is not to deny the complexity and competing nature of space nor to promote a false construction of isolated space (sectarianism) nor suggest a move to a dual space. There is no sacred space outside of the public world and any such suggestion is dualistic. Rather, as Cavanaugh argues, there are a "multiplicity of free spaces that are nonetheless fully public" and the way Christians live out the faithfully orientated story "transforms the way space is configured."⁷⁹ Therefore, it is not so much the space that should be the starting point but rather the *stories* shaping the space and resulting in different action that demand careful attention.

---

73. MacIntyre, *After Virtue*, 257.
74. Baker and Reader, *Entering the New Theological Space*, 3–5.
75. Cavanaugh, *Theopolitical Imagination*, 92.
76. Ibid.
77. Augustine, *The City of God against the Pagans*, 632.
78. Cavanaugh, *Theopolitical Imagination*, 84.
79. Ibid., 92–93.

One danger in framing the research question in terms of space or location could result in subsuming FBOs into civil society. As Cavanaugh argues, the notion of civil society as offering a space for the Church that is both "public" and "free" is flawed. In seeking to share space with civil society the Church will inevitably lose, "in part because the very distinction of public and private . . . is an instrument by which the state domesticates the Church."[80]

This process of "domestication" is not restricted to state-church relations. The neo-institutional school of organization theory has labeled the process "institutional isomorphism." As originally formulated,[81] institutional isomorphism identifies a process of increasing homogeneity in the forms and practices of organizations as they engage with other organizational fields where interaction, awareness, information, and structures of domination and coalition are shared. Proponents of neo-institutional theory argue that once disparate organizations engage in a common industry they become structured through organization-field forces such as market competition, state regulation, or professionalization and, often, emerge with strikingly similar forms and practices.[82] "Institutional isomorphism means convergence within organizational fields due to coercive, mimetic, and normative means of adaptation. Coercive isomorphism means adaptation due to formal or informal pressures or generalized expectations . . . Mimetic isomorphism points to the adaptation of technologies or organizational procedures . . . Normative isomorphism signifies adaptation mediated by processes of professionalization."[83] Such a process is particularly significant for an FBO engaging in health ministry in a contested and crowded space. The pressures upon FBOs have the potential to alter their *identity*.

There is multi-disciplinary interest in the development of identity and character.[84] A typical response to "domestication"—as Cavanaugh argues the Church is vulnerable through state domination[85]—is the assertion of identity. Although the identity of an FBO can morph under

---

80. Ibid., 54.
81. Di Maggio and Powell, "The Iron Cage Revisited," 70–74.
82. Swartz, "Secularization, Religion, and Isomorphism," 324.
83. Nagel, "Charitable Choices," 97.
84. Narvaez and Lapsley, *Personality, Identity, and Character*.
85. Cavanaugh, *Theopolitical Imagination*, 54.

pressure from external forces, it can also sustain its identity and character by drawing strength from outside itself. The process of institutional isomorphism is not inevitable. Smith and Sosin argue that if FBOs make conscious choices—regarding, for example, the sources of resources, the groups they partner with, the way they apply authority—they are able to shape organizational character. The process of shaping is dependent on the degree to which faith is coupled with the allocation of resources, the choice of partnerships, and the dominant sources of authority. The less the FBO is coupled to the faith community, the more the FBO will be coupled to secular society. "The tighter the coupling to religion, the more an agency's social organization reflects the demands of that religion."[86] Therefore, the choices made by FBOs are of critical importance. Excavating the underlying moral frameworks upon which FBOs make those choices is foundational to understanding the extent of coupling.

Although prioritizing space, location or identity was finally deemed an inadequate framework for this book, this is not to infer that they are not important factors requiring careful attention. Underplaying space and location can result in an inadequate grounding in reality—merely describing an orientation without linking it to concrete practice. This could allow FBOs to retreat into a sectarian position away from the contested reality within which health ministry for the poorest people must operate. Therefore, a significant portion of this book will describe and analyze the forces that inhabit space and recommend a place of "tension-dwelling"[87] for FBOs.

I finally settled on the following question: *"What characterizes faithfully orientated Salvation Army health ministry in the twenty-first century?"* It was clear the focus would be developing a faith-based future for Salvation Army health ministry—hence the terms "faithful" and "in the twenty-first century" provide a forward facing dynamic. The term "health ministry" rather than "health services" was chosen as it emphasizes the Christian practice of "ministry" rather than "services"—the latter suggesting a biomedical framework. This book argues that Christian engagement in health should not be redacted to "autonomy," "rights" or "service" but orientated on the basis of Christian soteriology understood

---

86. Smith and Sosin, "The Varieties of Faith-Related Agencies," 656.
87. Hauerwas and Coles, *Christianity, Democracy and the Radical Ordinary*, 15.

holistically as the work of redeeming persons who were created as "body-soul-in-relations."

My choice of orientation coupled with character should not be read as a rejection of the notion of space, place or identity but rather the assertion that a faithful identity capable of faithfully occupying space is dependent on priority being given to orientation or *telos*. Orientation is not merely a guiding light for occasional reference by the traveller. It is a rich, dense concept enabling the exploration and living out of the Christian story. It is indebted to Hellenistic philosophy promoted by Plato but, above all, Aristotle. In the past three decades, it received contemporary application in Alasdair MacIntyre's seminal book *After Virtue*. MacIntyre's central claim is that "it is only possible to understand the dominant moral culture of advanced modernity properly from a standpoint external to that culture."[88]

All moral life—and particularly Faith-Based Organizations as expressions of activities within particular moral traditions—requires a teleological conception of human existence towards somewhere, rather than forever being a movement between the "back and forth."[89] MacIntyre explains:

> Unless there is a *telos* which transcends the limited goods of practices by constituting the good of a whole human life, the good of a human life conceived as a unity, it will both be the case that a certain subversive arbitrariness will invade the moral life and that we shall be unable to specify the context of the virtues adequately. These two considerations are reinforced by a third: that there is at least one virtue recognized by the tradition which cannot be specified at all except with reference to the wholeness of a human life—the virtue of integrity or constancy. "Purity of heart" said Kierkegaard, "is to will one thing." This notion of singleness of purpose in a whole life can have no application unless that of a whole life does.[90]

MacIntyre's critique of the terms of moral debate in liberal democracies is foundational to this book. Although public debate in liberal democracies presumes everyone is speaking the same language, in fact, there are a number of operating discourses each using from lost moral

---

88. MacIntyre, *After Virtue*, vii.
89. Hauerwas, "A Retrospective Assessment of an 'Ethics of Character,'" 87.
90. MacIntyre, *After Virtue*, 203.

traditions, fragments that have become abstracted from a shared notion of what constitutes the good life and human flourishing. In the past, these notions were embodied in actual communities of discourse but, seduced by the "progress" of modernity, the moral traditions were disconnected from practice. These liberal democratic notions of the good life were given universality and generality and, in so doing, dispensed with the particularity of those traditions. "On the dominant liberal view government is to be neutral as between rival conceptions of the human good, yet, in fact, what liberalism promotes is a kind of institutional order that is inimical to the construction and sustaining of the types of communal relationship required for the best kind of human life."[91]

One outcome has been that the panoply of programs and initiatives proposed by liberal elite to solve the health problems of the poorest people amount "to a mass of conflicting universals competing for hegemony."[92] MacIntyre's corrective to the disruption of social relations is to encourage the regeneration of virtues through the everyday engagement of "plain persons"[93] in a variety of practices including "those making and sustaining families and households, schools, [and] clinics."[94]

This book seeks to identify an orientation for FBOs, which enables and sustains such "plain person" virtues and draws upon Christian theology as the foundational resource. It promotes an orientation for health ministry that prioritizes the cultivation of "healthy persons" enjoying faithful relationships and better health. As people continue to lose trust and hope in state and market-based health solutions, FBOs have an opportunity to promote a relational, holistic appreciation of human personhood. McIntyre's "plain person" virtues will be developed into a description of "healthy persons"—this book's recommended orientation for FBOs. The concept of "healthy persons" will be juxtaposed against the concept of the "autonomous rational individual" which currently orientates many secular health strategies. This book promotes an appreciation of "healthy persons" whose lives are soteriologically orientated and characterized by their relationship with God and their faithful presence in the

---

91. Ibid., xii.
92. Hovey, "Putting Truth to Practice," 170.
93. MacIntyre, *After Virtue*, xiii.
94. Ibid., xiii.

world. The *telos* of "healthy persons" transcends geographical, economic, and racial boundaries.

There are some disadvantages with using the term orientation. Those wishing to concentrate on the "effects" of truth without its non-public origins in the doctrine of a particular religion have used the term. Cavanaugh critiques the argument that theology can be appreciated for its contribution to the realm of public policy as long as its "basic orienting attitudes" are "translated into public policy by means of a social ethic, that is theories of justice, the state and so on, which cannot be derived directly from theology."[95] I reject any definition requiring a denuding of theological concepts in order to be understood by the "real world."

An "orientating concern" is not merely one theological concept among many, neither is it an abstract, conceptual perspective. It gains its relevance and significance from concrete practices. Cavanaugh argues the most fruitful way to dialogue with those outside of the Church is through "concrete practices that do not need translation into some putatively neutral language to be understood."[96] Cavanaugh proposes the liturgy as such a practice. However, few FBOs sustain their orientation by careful attention to liturgy—and The Salvation Army certainly does not. Bretherton argues for contemporary politics to be attentive to existing practices such as hospitality and listening.[97] This book is promoting health ministry as such a practice. The priority in all these practices is to develop resilient relationships of friendship. As Hauerwas argues: "Christians are a people who believe that the many narratives that constitute our lives finally have the *telos* of making us God's friends and, in the process, making us friends with one another and even friends with our own life."[98]

To summarize: In seeking a faithful orientation for Salvation Army health ministry there is no intention to underplay the complexity, realities, and conflicting priorities of the task. State, market, and communitarian forces dominate health care space and identity around the world. As Salvation Army health ministries operate in more than 120 countries, any orientation needs to resonate in a multiplicity of contexts. I contend a common, articulated *telos* is possible and can result in more faithful

---

95. Cavanaugh, *Theopolitical Imagination*, 61.

96. Ibid., 94.

97. Bretherton, *Christianity and Contemporary Politics*, 220.

98. Hauerwas, *Sanctify Them in the Truth*, 103.

Salvation Army health ministry around the globe.[99] FBOs should not presume to speak the same language as organizations that rely on operating discourses based on fragments abstracted from communities of discourse. Any presumption of common language threatens the integrity, orientation, and ultimately the effectiveness of FBOs and other groups.

BOOK OVERVIEW

Chapter 2 begins working through Swinton and Mowat's model of practical theology[100] by describing and analyzing state and market "solutions" for improving the health of the poorest people. Sustaining a long-term faithful orientation is only possible, I argue, if FBOs are alert to the pressures from the competing narratives for "good health" from state and market. Karl Polanyi's 1944 analysis of the economic and social changes following the Industrial Revolution argues that social relations became disembedded by a dominant market economy.[101] Polanyi's critique of market domination aided by the liberal state identified the dynamic of disrupted social relations that is particularly damaging to the health of the poorest people. Polanyi's framework enables an analysis of the contemporary actions of the state and market upon the health of the poorest people. This description is enriched by field reflections from India (where market forces are a major influence in shaping health care provision) and Zambia (where the state directed health care provision is dominant). The concept of the "autonomous rational individual" is identified as serving market and state "solutions" for commodified and instrumental ends. However, the "autonomous rational individual" is critiqued as a flawed *telos*.

Chapter 3 continues with Step Two of the practical theological reflection process by describing and analyzing the context of FBO health ministry. The state and the market are not the only spheres influencing the health of the poorest people. Other spheres may be less formal but are still influential. Community-centric, Third Sector and FBO "solutions" are described and analyzed, enhanced by field reflections from Papua

---

99. Limited reference is made to Salvation Army health ministry in economically developed countries due to my focus on improving the health of the poorest people in the world. However, they face challenges in sustaining teleological faithfulness.

100. Swinton and Mowat, *Practical Theology and Qualitative Research*, 94–97.

101. Polanyi, *The Great Transformation*, 45–80.

New Guinea and Netherlands. Adalbert Evers' framework for appreciating the role of the Third Sector as part of a mixed welfare system—otherwise made up of the market, state, and the informal sphere of households and families—highlights the significance of the process of institutional isomorphism. Evers notes the importance of *telos* in sustaining the character of FBOs and recommends a "civilized culture of conflict"[102] against the isomorphic tendencies of the market and state.

The terms upon which partnerships are developed and "common ground" is established and sustained are of critical importance to this thesis. There are two significant risks for an FBO—assimilation or isolation. Chapter 3 analyses recent literature on FBO context, typologies, and three frameworks—dignity and rights,[103] social justice,[104] and role and function[105]—for establishing "common ground" between FBOs and wider society. The analysis concludes that "common ground" should be sought, not based on a shared *telos*, but in a spirit of respectful tension dwelling based on mutual interest. Sustaining this position is difficult, however; resilient relationships are key and are aided by FBOs contributing to what Bretherton identifies as the "building blocks of a more complex space that inhibits the totalizing, monopolistic thrust of the modern market and state that seek to instrumentalize and commodify persons and the relationships between them."[106]

The final section of Chapter 3 seeks to recover a faithful orientation for the institutions of clinics, hospitals, and congregations so they have the capacity to resist the forces of the market and state and provide spaces for health and healing. The history and current context is described and analyzed. It is argued that faith-based institutions—clinics, hospitals, and congregations—should be places of refuge from the forces of instrumentalism and commodification. Proposals to abandon health work to bio-medical professionals are criticized. This thesis argues that faithfully orientated clinic-hospitals and churches offer an important "institutional space" for poor and marginalized people; an anchor, a non-pecuniary

---

102. Evers, "Part of the Welfare Mix," 167.
103. Smith and Sosin, "The Varieties of Faith-Related Agencies," 665.
104. Olivier, "In Search of Common Ground," 173.
105. Bane et al., *Taking Faith Seriously*, 8.
106. Bretherton, "A Postsecular Politics?," 9.

space where people of all faiths (and none) can strive together towards better health.

Chapter 4 continues with the process of contextual and cultural analysis by describing and analyzing Salvation Army practice of health ministry and other social services. The writing of two influential Salvation Army officers, William Booth and Philip Needham, are reviewed. A number of issues in Salvation Army theology and practice are identified as requiring theological reflection in order to sustain a faithful *telos* and, thereby, improve health ministry for the poorest people. These include a theologically based understanding of personhood; the relationship between the Spirit, the church, and the world; the importance of habits and practices in sustaining a faithful *telos*; as well as the contribution of clinic-hospitals, congregations, and other community groups to the task of improving the health of the poorest people.

Chapter 5 moves to Stage Three of the model—theological reflection—and responds to issues raised in the preceding chapters by reflecting on the practices of faith-based health ministry in the light of scripture and tradition.[107] This theological reflection is structured around the key scriptural themes of creation, fall, and redemption. First, a reflection on the created nature of personhood and an understanding of "health" contributes to the development of the concept of "healthy persons." Personhood, as understood in Christian theology, includes rational (body-soul) as well as relational (persons-in-relation) dimensions. Health is not conceptualized as a goal of itself but, is a means for more faithful participation of the people of God in the work of the Kingdom. Therefore, "healthy persons" is an eschatological appreciation of people created as integrated "body-soul-in-relations," who do not overvalue or undervalue their individuality, but understand themselves and other humans as unique gifts, made in the image of God with capacity for relationships. This chapter argues that "healthy persons" develop a particular relationship with their immediate locality (family, friends, neighborhood, nation) as well as sustaining a relationship with all humanity. However, "healthy persons" living in the *saeculum* are fallen, fractured, and in ongoing need of redemption which is possible through the work of Christ, perfected by the power of the Holy Spirit and sustained by institutions, habits, and practices of faithful people.

---

107. Swinton and Mowat, *Practical Theology and Qualitative Research*, 95.

An appreciation of the impact of the Fall is developed in a review of modern medical practice. The western biomedical model of medicine is critiqued for offering an alternative soteriology that promises far more than it can deliver. The work of Stanley Hauerwas is foundational in appreciating the responsibility of the Church to present the world with an alternative understanding of health, healing, and living with disease. In the third section—redemption—Hauerwas's conception of the institution of the Church and its practices are reflected upon. The practice of faithful presence amid tension dwelling is proposed as a key characteristic of "healthy persons" and of FBOs engaged in health ministry. The resources to sustain faithfully orientated FBOs in places of tension dwelling require the life, practices, and habits of the worshipping community. By seeking a shared *telos* and fostering a common character, FBOs, clinics, and congregations can occupy a distinct space and, in doing so, faithfully engage in their fragmented and unhealthy world.

Chapter 6, the concluding chapter, undertakes Stage Four of the practical theology model—formulating revised practice. Characteristics of faithfully orientated Salvation Army health ministry are drawn out of the preceding discussion. The characteristics of *movement* for the development of *"healthy persons"* formed and sustained by the *habits and practices* of worshipping congregations in the power of the Spirit is proposed. These "healthy persons" work together to support clinic-hospitals, households, and other institutions and groups with *theologically reflective* ways of working resulting in the transformation of *social relations* as God intends. The chapter includes examples of Salvation Army health ministry in Bolivia, Ghana, and Kenya where the characteristics of such ministry are evident in contemporary practice. The conclusion includes practical recommendations for more faithful Salvation Army health ministry in the twenty-first century and wider implications for other FBOs.

2

Health for the Poorest People: The Contribution of the State and the Market

THIS CHAPTER BEGINS THE second step in the practical theological reflection process by "entering into dialogue with other sources of knowledge which will help us develop a deeper understanding of the situation."[1] Improving the health of the poorest people requires FBOs to engage with a number of players operating in the health care system such as governments, markets, households, communities, not-for-profit organizations, and other faith-based organizations who operate from various faith-bases. The next three chapters describe and analyze the context within which FBOs operate with specific reference to The Salvation Army. This chapter begins by examining the two dominant players—the state and the market.

ANALYZING THE SPHERES CONTESTING THE SPACE

The two dominant forces influencing health care around the world are, without doubt, the state and the market. Karl Polanyi highlights the impact of the market and state on the health of the poorest people and their social relations.[2]

---

1. Swinton and Mowat, *Practical Theology and Qualitative Research*, 95–96.
2. Polanyi, *The Great Transformation*.

State and Market—Karl Polanyi's Analysis

Before the upheavals of the Industrial Revolution, Polanyi argues, markets were nothing more than "accessories of economic life."[3] After the Industrial Revolution, all transactions received a monetary value. Not just goods produced for sale on a market but also, what he terms, "fictitious" commodities such as land, labor, and goods are expected to behave in the same way. Polanyi argues this is a mistaken assumption resulting in "an economy directed by market prices and nothing but market prices."[4]

This assumption led, after the great transformation of the industrial revolution, to markets receiving priority over every other sphere—politics, religion, and social relations. Polanyi critiques the theory of market liberalism that developed in the nineteenth century and challenges its core belief that human society should be subordinated to self-regulating markets. Polanyi argues: "The control of the economic system by the market is of overwhelming consequence to the whole organization of society: it means no less than the running of society as an adjunct to the market. Instead of economy being embedded in social relations, social relations are embedded in the economy."[5]

Polanyi argues it is morally wrong to treat human beings as objects whose price is determined entirely by the market.[6] He also argues the faith placed in the self-regulatory capacity of the market is misplaced. Instability caused by free markets is inevitable and will demand intervention by the state to prevent societal breakdown.[7] This is Polanyi's "double movement thesis" which Gareth Dale defines as "the commodification of land, labor, and money that results in social disintegration, compelling society to protect itself by delegating the state to regulate fictitious commodities."[8] Inevitably, significant state intervention is required to impose and sustain the global market system.[9] Therefore, the notion that markets can be self-regulating is flawed and, Polanyi argues, they should not be able to pretend they are. He asserts that the proponents of the

---

3. Ibid., 71.
4. Ibid., 45.
5. Ibid., 60.
6. Block, *Introduction to the Great Transformation*, xxv.
7. Polanyi, *The Great Transformation*, 70–80.
8. Dale, *Karl Polanyi*, 71.
9. Polanyi, *The Great Transformation*, 66–70.

free-market doctrine are promoting a "utopian project: something that cannot exist."[10]

Polanyi argues that market liberalism makes demands on ordinary people that are not sustainable.[11] For example, the periodic, dramatic fluctuations in the commodity market are damaging to farmers, small business people, and low-paid workers. As the impact of commodification driven by market forces causes social disruption—as they inevitably do—society demands the state intervenes to repair the damage. For example, the state intervenes in the money markets to avoid the damage of inflation and deflation; in the use of land through planning permission and agricultural subsidies; and, critically for this book, the state intervenes to manipulate social relations often at the cost of the poorest people in the service of the liberal market. Fred Block, writing 60 years after Polanyi, identifies contemporary risks from free markets: "In every corner of the globe militant movements—often intermixed with religious fundamentalism—are poised to take advantage of the economic and social shocks of globalization."[12]

The care of sick people reveals particular tensions in the functioning of the market-state. Issues that are a priority in social relationships like life, health, and death, tend to be commodified by the market. To put it bluntly, a sick person is not useful to the state as an instrument or to the market as a commodity—they are simply a burden. The poorest people are often the sickest and the least able to pay for market-provided health services. When priority is given to deregulated market forces, the "unhealthy poor" become an unattractive problem.

Polanyi offers a nuanced argument beyond the simplistic labels of capitalist, socialist or Marxist[13] and presents "a coherent analysis of the institutional arrangements governing the production, exchange, and valuation of goods other than by the market system."[14] He accepts the role of markets but demands conscious limits are placed on the freedom of the market to bring about a re-embedding of the market within social relations. Dale describes Polanyi's countermovement as a "heuristic that

10. Block, *Introduction to the Great Transformation*, xxiv.
11. Polanyi, *The Great Transformation*, 136–40.
12. Block, *Introduction to the Great Transformation*, xxxv.
13. Ibid., xxix.
14. Dale, *Karl Polanyi*, 141.

refers to the way in which when the self-regulating market undermines the security of their livelihoods, human beings look to political ideas and organizations that claim to defend society against market excesses."[15] Bretherton identifies the contemporary example of health and safety regulations as a "counter-movement" by the state on the market in order to protect employees, customers, and wider society.[16] I am proposing that FBOs understand their contribution to improving the health of the poorest people as a "counter-movement" against the commodification of health care. FBO health care for the poorest people can be enhanced if it is orientated by the importance of re-embedding economic relations within social relations by connecting people (rich and poor; healthy and sick) into an "intentional moral relationship, which recognizes that my continued wellbeing is related to the wellbeing of all."[17]

Polanyi's analysis of economic theory provides important insights for The Salvation Army and other FBOs with his analysis of the impact and influence of markets on the lives and relationships of ordinary people—particularly the economically disadvantaged.[18] In turn, this is an important consideration for FBOs in determining the nature of their relations with state and market forces. FBOs need to be wary of becoming agents of instrumentalization or commodification and support "counter-movements" that enhance the health of people—particularly the poorest.

Contemporary Reflections on Polanyi

Polanyi did not get it completely right and he incorrectly predicted the end of the self-regulating market in 1944.[19] No doubt Polanyi would be surprised at the resilience of "faith in the market" in many parts of the world—even post the current financial and banking global crisis. Despite evidence to the contrary, the belief persists that "if individuals and firms are given maximum freedom to pursue their economic self-interest, the global marketplace will make everyone better off."[20] This confidence is

---

15. Ibid., 220.
16. Bretherton, *Christianity and Contemporary Politics*, 185.
17. Ibid.
18. MacIntyre, Hauerwas, Evers and Bretherton acknowledge the influence of Karl Polanyi on their work.
19. Polanyi, *The Great Transformation*, 148.
20. Block, *Introduction to the Great Transformation*, xxxiii.

particularly misplaced when it is applied to solutions for improving the health of the poorest people.[21] Polanyi's critique is used against the promoters of the Washington Consensus,[22] neo-liberal globalization[23] and in defense of the national state.[24]

The similarities between Polanyi's descriptions of late nineteenth and early twentieth-century European conditions and the challenges facing developing countries today were highlighted in recent academic research.[25] Historically, communities, and economies in the developing world were embedded in society through concepts of reciprocity, exchange, and redistribution but are now experiencing rapid transformation from the forces of economic globalization. Currently, many millions of rural people in the developing world are losing access to the land and do not have property rights. Urban dwellers do not fare better with a lack of secure employment destabilizing society—due to increasingly informal employment practices; increasing competition and deregulation keeps wages low and unemployment high—coupled with access to health services, water, sanitation, and education being patchy and expensive.[26]

Polanyi's analysis informed research into the migration of women carers from the Indian state of Kerela, leaving children and family to meet the demand for carers in western countries.[27] The market demands of the north indirectly erode the social solidarities of the south. The loss of mothers from developing world communities across the globe will significantly weaken the capacity of those countries to develop—economically, politically, and socially.[28] This research resonates with my reflections on

---

21. For a detailed assessment of Polanyi's contribution to the contemporary debate see Dale, *Karl Polanyi*, 207–50.

22. The 'Washington Consensus' is a label attached to the ideological agenda of neo-liberalism for which economists such as Friedman and von Hayek were noted along with the economic programs implemented by Reagan and Thatcher in the 1980s. The main goal of the Washington Consensus was the reactivation and promotion of economic growth in Latin America, yet precluded any concern for redistribution. See Montiel, "Incompleteness of Post-Washington Consensus."

23. Silver and Arrighi, "Polanyi's 'Double Movement,'" 325.

24. Holmwood, "Three Pillars of Welfare State Theory," 23.

25. "Development's Invisible Hands," Development Studies Association Conference, 2008, London.

26. Stewart, "Relaxing the Shackles," 2.

27. Isaksen et al., "Global Care Crisis," 409.

28. Ibid., 410.

market inducements encouraging The Salvation Army in India to train young women as nurses primarily to secure their passage out of India to work in the Gulf States, USA or Europe.

In summary, Polanyi's analysis of market and state spheres of operation and influence is helpful in describing and analyzing the contemporary context within which the poorest people live—and become sick—and within which FBOs operate. Counter movements can restrain the market and promote the value of people in social relationships. This book promotes faith-based health ministry—characterized by practices such as hospitality and listening—as a counter-movement capable of resisting the instrumentalizing and commodifying forces of the market-state.

FIELD REFLECTIONS

In light of Polanyi's analysis of the impact of the market and state on social relations, I turn to field reflections from India and Zambia to highlight the challenges poor people face in accessing health care. These reflections enrich the cultural and contextual analysis step of the practical theological reflection model.

India

Like many Christian missionary enterprises, the development of Salvation Army hospitals in India occurred in the first half of the twentieth century,[29] associated with the British colonial period.[30] Between 1900 and 1940, The Salvation Army opened 12 large hospitals in India.[31] These institutions were, for many years, run by Western missionaries and proved popular

---

29. The first Christian missionaries arrived in India in 1727 but it was after 1835—when English replaced Persian as the official language—that Christian education and social services in India expanded. Although they now represent only 2 percent of the national population, Christians are still perceived to exercise significant social influence in India through schools and hospitals. See Bano and Nair, "Faith Based Organizations in South Asia," 14.

30. Ibid., 22.

31. The annual statistics published in 1941 by Salvation Army International Headquarters gives a total of 62 hospitals and 32 dispensaries, of which 17 were in the USA, 4 in Canada, 12 in India, 4 in Australia, 6 in New Zealand and 8 in the then Dutch East Indies (Indonesia). There were nearly 200,000 inpatients (Williams, 2009, p69). By 2008, all of the hospitals in USA, Canada, Australia and New Zealand were no longer under Salvation Army management. See Williams, *Every Army Needs an Ambulance Corps*, 23ff.

with local people due to their quality of care—subsidized by donations from overseas. The missionary administrators were able to access funding from the colonial government to develop the facilities and fund the provision of services. Large plots of land in small towns were allocated to The Salvation Army and a mission compound was developed typically including a hospital and an education program (primary, secondary, and/or nurse training school) and a corps (church). Some compounds also had agricultural projects. The missionaries lived on the compound and built a community within the walls.

By the time I commenced this research in 2007, The Salvation Army had no western missionaries working in India.[32] The numbers declined since the 1970s and by the 1990s only a handful of westerners were serving in Indian hospitals. I made eight visits to India while researching this book and visited all six Salvation Army territories.[33] There are currently nine Salvation Army hospitals in India and I visited all of them in 2008. They are scattered across India from Dhariwal in the northwest on the Pakistan border to Nagercoil near the southeastern tip of the country. Most of these are large general hospitals and all are struggling—to some extent—with too few patients and too many staff; pre-1980 management systems; old buildings and ancient equipment. Several of the hospitals in India are technically bankrupt and paying some staff salaries four or five months late.[34]

The aspirations and expectations of Indian patients are changing rapidly. Most wish to see a specialist doctor for relatively minor ailments and are willing to pay for costly, and often unnecessary, tests. There are as many as 30 specialist doctors linked to some Salvation Army hospitals—on a part-time basis—with a tendency to refer patients to their small, self-owned, private, specialist hospitals if the patient is able to pay. This drives up the cost of treatment, skims off the profitable patients—leaving

---

32. The term 'missionaries' was discontinued in the early 1990s and 'reinforcement personnel' is now used. Indian visa restrictions prohibit The Salvation Army appointing reinforcement personnel to India at present.

33. The Salvation Army in India is divided into six territories with headquarters in Delhi, Mumbai, Chennai, Aizawl, Maharajanagar and Thiruvananthapuram. I visited all nine Indian hospitals, many community-based health programs and churches in urban and rural locations across India.

34. The doctors were paid on time and in full as they would leave if they did not get paid. The general staff were however made to wait until the administrator could raise the cash.

The Salvation Army with the "unprofitable poor"—and reduces the provision of integrated, holistic patient care.

Indian government regulations and constitutional court guarantees appear unable to resist the ravages of the market. A reporter for *The Hindustan Times* highlights incidents at government hospitals where pregnant women have been denied treatment due to their inability to pay. These commercially driven actions have resulted in maternal and child deaths with mothers delivering babies in cars and under trees just outside the hospital gates. These incidents occur despite an Indian Supreme Court ruling that hospitals cannot refuse admission and treatment to critically ill or emergency patients on any grounds.[35] A review of Public Health literature highlighted similar trends. The commodification of health care inhibits poor people from gaining access to health services and negatively affects the quality and cost of medical care.[36] The commercialization of health services and medicalization through adherence to biomedical health approaches is resulting in poor quality care across South Asia.[37]

Christians are a minority in India. While India projects itself as a modern, secular state, there is a strong perception of state bias towards Hindus and against Christians and Muslims.[38] Indian Salvationists repeatedly expressed a sense of disadvantage and discrimination. Coupled with the widespread, persistent application of the caste system, this leaves almost all Indian Salvationists (predominately from the lowest caste groups) unable to move beyond the poor and marginalized sections of Indian society. Indian Salvationists often blamed the decline in clinical care and patient numbers on a lack of dedicated doctors.[39] With the departure of the missionary doctors—who generally had a strong sense of vocation and could access donations from home—their replacement Indian doctors often face large student and dowry debts, unrealistic family expectations, and little access to overseas donor funds. Indian Salvationists are unreasonable in contrasting the dedication of local doctors with that

---

35. Jaya Shroff Bhalla, "Hospitals 'Blatantly' Flout Supreme Court Ruling."
36. Das and Hammer, "Money for Nothing," 2.
37. Shaikh et al., "Health Care and Public Health in South Asia," 143.
38. Bano and Nair, "Faith Based Organizations in South Asia," 1545–62.

39. The doctors also often expressed frustration at the poor quality of administration and leadership given by the Salvation Army leaders. This often seemed to be a reasonable criticism.

of the missionaries. The pressures upon the Indian doctors to conform to market and societal expectations are enormous.

Almost all Salvation Army hospital managers and doctors in India recommended greater commercialization of Salvation Army health programs. This was justified on the premise of making profits from the rich to subsidize the care of the poor. This has historically been a means of sustaining Salvation Army health ministry as noted by Harry Williams, a Salvation Army officer doctor who served for many years in India: "By 1950 there was a total of 1,000 hospital beds in India still supported in the same way; the income generated by the high quality of its services, which drew a stream of paying patients, subsidizing those unable to pay."[40]

I observed Salvation Army administrators applying convoluted charging systems based on different classes of patient care. Indian Government health policy forced this move towards commercialization by providing almost no support to Salvation Army hospitals[41] and regulating them as part of the private sector. Unlike many African countries, where the state funds mission hospitals to provide services on behalf of the state, there are few similar financial grants in India. A visit to a Catholic hospital in Indonesia and a Church of South India hospital in Kerela revealed other denominations also struggling to succeed with a hospital financing model attempting to provide health care for the poorest on the back of profits from wealthier patients. It is difficult to make adequate profits due to competition in terms of quality and cost from commercial health-care providers.

I noted tensions between doctors, nurses, and Salvation Army officer administrators partly due to a lack of financial investment in hospital infrastructure, poor administrative decisions, and understandable frustration at declining standards. A number of doctors were manipulating the services for their financial benefit. However, simply replacing the administrator or the doctors is not the answer—the context has changed and the model of large, multi-specialist general hospitals run by churches is no longer sustainable no matter who is in charge.

The main response of The Salvation Army in India to the decline in patient revenue has been to expand the number and size of nursing training schools. Salvation Army nurse education is very popular as it

40. Williams, *Every Army Needs an Ambulance Corps*, xvi.

41. There are a few examples of district health teams working with Salvation Army health teams with vaccination programs but there is generally little collaboration.

offers an escape route from discrimination based on caste, gender, and faith through emigration to wealthier countries such as the Gulf States, Europe, and North America. Therefore, parents are prepared to pay fees to secure a recognized qualification and this gives hospital administrators a vital source of income. However, improving the health of the poorest people in India is not helped by a generation of women emigrating. Additionally, the quality of nurse training is inadequate with few patients in the hospitals making it impossible for students to gain adequate practical experience.

Despite all the faults and failings, Salvationists in India do not want their hospitals to close. They believe health institutions give The Salvation Army and the wider Christian community, an important opportunity for ministry. Some people of other faiths view non-institutional Christian health ministry—such as community or home visits—with suspicion, fearing they are a front for evangelism. The fastest growing Salvation Army community-based programs in India are self-help groups responding to poverty—particularly among women—through the creation of savings groups and income-generation activities. These initiatives could be an effective counter-movement to the ravages of commodification of social relations in India but the leaders struggle to articulate a theological rationale for these programs and are at risk of merely aping the market.

This Indian vignette has illustrated the complexity of health ministry in a context impacted by factors such as the colonial legacy, ongoing religious, and caste prejudice, secularization, professionalization, and, in particular, market forces. The number of complex issues facing Salvation Army decision-makers in India is overwhelming and current responses are incoherent and fragmented.

Zambia

Unlike India where the market dominates the health care sector, in Zambia the state is the main actor.[42] In a country with 72 different languages and more than 100 tribal groups with the consequent risk of factionalism, the nation-state is viewed as a unifying force. Being a "good Zambian" has become a widely accepted social norm since the birth of the nation in 1964. Christianity's relationship with the state was formalized when the former

---

42. My wife and I served in Zambia from 1996 to 2000 working at the Salvation Army hospital at Chikankata. I made further visits in 2002, 2007, 2008 and 2011.

President Frederick Chiluba declared Zambia a "Christian country" in 1992. Chikankata Mission[43] in southern Zambia was established by The Salvation Army in 1946 and developed a close relationship with the state that continues to the present day.

In 2007, Chikankata Health Services had a financial turnover of more than US$ 4 million. It comprises a 125 bed hospital, community health program for 90,000 people, oversees 5 rural health centers on behalf of the district health office; has a nursing training school for 175 enrolled nurses and midwives plus a biomedical college for 90 students. Chikankata has been the trendsetter for international Salvation Army health ministry attracting more than US$1.1 million from donor funding for community health work. In 2007, the Government of Zambia funding to Chikankata Health Services accounted for more than 50 percent of its income by direct payment for staff salaries and running cost grants. Most of this money comes from western government donations into the government health budget and as such is vulnerable to the vagaries of western donor priorities. However, Chikankata Health Services still struggles to access sufficient funding for activities not popular with donors such as in-patient costs and infrastructural maintenance.

Like many African countries, Zambia has undergone a number of political and economic transitions over recent decades from colonial rule (1890 to 1964), to a centrally planned command economy under Kenneth Kaunda (1964 to 1991), to a more market driven economy under several Movement for Multiparty Democracy governments (1991 to 2011). In the past 35 years, the Zambian economy has shrunk significantly resulting in a corresponding decline in state health expenditure. Using 1995 prices for comparative purposes, the government budget for health fell from US$29 per capita in 1970 to US$2.60 in 1998. The Government of Zambia with involvement from western agencies such as the World Bank and IMF has attempted a number of structural reforms to improve Zambian health services.

---

43. Chikankata Mission is located 31km from the main tar road in a very rural location. In addition to the health programs based at Chikankata, The Salvation Army also runs a 800-pupil boarding high school; a radio station; the divisional headquarters for Salvation Army churches (corps). The mission has built its own dam, water purification plant, internal electricity reticulation system and is responsible for maintaining 300 houses for the staff. In effect, The Salvation Army is running a small town with a population in excess of 2,500 people.

The Zambian government's health vision since 1992, is to "provide Zambians with equity of access to cost effective and quality health care as close to the family as possible." Steps have been taken by the Ministry of Health—under close watch from the donor community—to improve community participation in decision-making; reform large hospitals; improve the health funding by adopting a sector wide approach seeking to bring all health funding together in a joint sectoral framework. The reforms have not succeeded as planned: decentralization has had little impact—positive or negative—on services;[44] the structures established to improve community participation have had little impact;[45] attempts to increase revenue by introducing patient user-fees and health insurance have failed and, in fact, often made the situation worse for the poorest people[46] large Zambian hospitals have not reformed;[47] and the sector wide approach to funding is not fully effective.[48]

Improving primary health care requires the difficult political decision to reduce funding to hospitals. Health academics, strategists, and donors often demonize hospitals, particularly in sub-Saharan Africa. One describes them as the "consumers of excessive resources, magnets for patients whose needs would be better met elsewhere and as inefficient dinosaurs whose activities should be reined in."[49] There is some justification for such a view. Three central hospitals in Zambia together with 19 second-level referral hospitals (of which Chikankata is one) consumed approximately 40 percent of the Zambian health budget in 1998.[50]

The Zambian government attempted to address this problem in the 1990s with a hospitals reform program based on two principles—decentralization of authority and greater exposure to market forces.[51]

44. Bossert and Beauvais, "Decentralization of Health Systems in Ghana, Zambia, Uganda and the Philippines," 14.

45. Macwan'gi and Ngwengwe, "Effectiveness of District Health Boards," 72.

46. Ekman, "Catastrophic Health Payments and Health Insurance," 312. Van Der Geest et al., "User Fees and Drugs," 59.

47. Hanson et al., "Towards Improving Hospital Performance in Uganda and Zambia," 74.

48. Chansa et al., "Exploring Swap's Contribution," 244.

49. Hanson et al., "Towards Improving Hospital Performance in Uganda and Zambia," 74.

50. Ibid.

51. Blas and Limbambala, "The Challenge of Hospitals in Health Sector Reform," 30. Hanson et al., "Towards Improving Hospital Performance in Uganda and Zambia," 92.

However, there was a reaction against greater exposure to market forces with members of parliament opposing a reduction in funding to secondary and tertiary level hospitals. While this saved the large hospitals, the vital expansion of primary health care services could not be funded and was shelved. The Zambian Parliament, in terms of Polanyi's thesis, has to some extent, resisted the unbridled application of market forces—in the guise of western donor pressure—but this did not lead to improved health services.

The Christian mission hospitals, clinics, and community based health services provide approximately 30 percent of all Zambian health services.[52] The state significantly contributes to the funding of mission health services and, in turn, the Churches Health Association of Zambia (CHAZ), which acts as a coordinating body, represents Zambian mission hospitals and clinics at the Ministry of Health.[53] In 1996, a Memorandum of Understanding was signed between the Minister of Health and CHAZ aiming to provide for greater alignment between FBO and government structures, by agreeing that management boards administered by the church would have the same powers as those established under the National Health Services Act, 1995.[54]

I was present at negotiations in the late 1990s regarding the Memorandum of Understanding between CHAZ and the Ministry of Health. Despite regular protestations from the church leaders about resisting state influence in the running of mission hospitals—retaining the

52. The Churches Health Association of Zambia (CHAZ) was established in 1970 to serve as an umbrella organization of church health institutions and community-based organizations. CHAZ now comprises of 129 members, which together account for 59 percent of health care coverage in the rural areas of Zambia and 30 percent of the health care in the country as a whole. The extensive CHAZ network includes 32 hospitals, 68 health care clinics and 26 community-based organizations. CHAZ's role expanded rapidly in recent years when it received US$50 million in direct Global Fund financing through 2008. See The Capacity Project, "Working with Faith-Based Organizations to Strengthen Human Resources for Health."

53. Christian Health Associations are a significant player in African heath services. For example, the Christian Health Association of Kenya (CHAK), founded in 1982, covers 24 hospitals, 43 health centers, 298 dispensaries and 51 church health programs and includes more than a dozen denominations. CHAK members are providing about 40 percent of Kenya's health services. Similarly, the Christian Health Association of Malawi (CHAM), founded in 1966, comprises 28 hospitals and 125 health centers and its member FBOs provide about 37 percent of the country's health services. Ibid.

54. Hanson et al., "Towards Improving Hospital Performance in Uganda and Zambia," 85.

right of the church to discipline staff, appoint senior staff, retain the spiritual character of the hospitals, etc—Zambian Christian leaders seem keen to embrace government health priorities as far as possible. Partnership arrangements such as the Memorandum of Understanding between CHAZ and the MOH were presented to the hospitals with the understanding they will increase autonomy and local decision-making but, one of the western consultants driving the reforms admitted the outcome would be different: "By integrating NGO budgets and plans into the overall MOH framework, autonomous hospital policies can help to harmonize standards and practices among public and private facilities. Ironically, this will actually reduce the autonomy enjoyed by NGO facilities."[55]

It is unclear whether African governments view the churches' involvement in health services as merely a remnant of the continent's colonial history—to be endured for the present until the market-state is able to replace FBOs—or if they value the contribution FBOs can make in resisting the excess of the commodification of medicine and the strengthening of social relations. This is a pressing issue across Africa. Faith-based health programs in Zambia—as in Ghana, Tanzania, Uganda, and Zimbabwe—provide up to 40 percent of the nation's health care through mission hospitals and clinics.[56] However, the recently published African Health Strategy (2007 to 2015) only mentions "faith" once in 30 pages (in a footnote on p23) and collapses the faith contribution into the wider definition of "civil society" while "traditional healers" received half a page of strategic commitment.[57]

An analysis of the relationship between mission hospital, local churches, and community groups provides additional complexification. The long-term Salvation Army institutional presence at Chikankata has resulted in the highest density of Salvation Army churches (corps) in Zambia within a 50-mile radius of the mission. Although Chikankata Mission is a source of pride for members of The Salvation Army, the complexity of the relationships and the resource demands of Chikankata Mission have inhibited the maturation of other Salvation Army ministries across Zambia. For example, there have been disagreements over the methods used by public health practitioners in working with

---

55. Ibid., 90.

56. Olivier et al., "Working in a Bounded Field of Unknowing,"

57. African Conference of Health Ministers, "African Health Strategy—2007 to 2015," 15.

the Chikankata community. Health workers do not always find it easy to work with church leaders and, therefore, prefer to develop community links through the traditional leadership structure (represented by chief and headmen). Often the church is by-passed—or given notional acknowledgment—by public health workers even when employed by a FBO. This tension between FBO health programs and church congregations is becoming increasingly complicated across Africa by the willingness of western donors to pay community volunteers for participating in health programs. This is disempowering the church-based groups—who are rarely paid—and threatens a decline in the voluntary work done by church members.

This Zambian vignette highlights the influence external donors have on the state and church; and the impact that state policy and professional practice has on the ministry of the Church. The Zambian case study identifies some of the effects of professionalizing health care and the impact this has on individuals in their community, some of whom will also be church members. Tensions in the relationship between a large faith based institution and the local congregation have been noted.[58]

These two field reflections have noted examples of countries adopting state-centric responses to the health of the poorest people (Zambia) as well as more market-centric responses (India). The next two sections of this chapter triangulate the field experiences with literature promoting state-centric and market-centric responses. This will develop a fuller appreciation of the cultural and contextual factors impacting the health of the poorest people.

STATE-CENTRIC RESPONSES

This next section does not attempt to offer a detailed reflection on the contribution of the state in improving the health of the poorest people. Rather it briefly identifies some of the pressures upon the state affecting relationships with FBOs in developing countries. The starting point is not to deny or undervalue the importance of a functioning state in all countries. Public health disasters in failed states illustrate the importance of the state in the task of improving the health of the

---

58. I noted similar levels of attachment and frustration in congregations relating to large hospitals among Salvation Army church members in Zimbabwe, India and Indonesia.

poorest people. However, the state—in developing countries—rarely has a strong and robust capacity to deliver health care due to it being reshaped by multiple forces acting simultaneously: "From above, the state is actively constrained by agreements promoted by international agencies and by the power of multinational corporations. From within, the state is being reshaped by increasing trends toward marketization and by problems of corruption. From below, the state's role is being diminished by the expansion of decentralization and by the rising influence of non-governmental organizations."[59]

Therefore, FBOs need to be alert to the forces shaping the health landscape and respond accordingly. Firstly, foreign government donors are often very influential on national government policy. Although western donors and international agencies acknowledge the importance of strong national health policy, the recipient nations are obliged—even pressurized—to adopt "approved" approaches in order to receive funding. The Paris Declaration on Aid Effectiveness "emphasized the harmonization of donor procedures and the alignment of initiatives with local policies and systems."[60] It called for government-led sector-wide approaches in health services and donors being "explicitly linked to national health plans and underpinned by strong performance-based principles."[61] This trend towards harmonization—with increased state-led centralization—threatens the space available for FBOs and reduces grassroots participation.

An Australia government policy document suggests a helpful way forward by rejecting a dogmatic insistence on centralized ways of delivering health through prioritizing "outputs, outcomes, and impacts rather than focus on the process of aid interventions outcomes."[62] The acknowledgement by Government policy makers of the importance of *process* is most welcome. A key recommendation of this book will be for FBOs—and governments—to give greater attention to the process of building and sustaining of relationships with the poorest people. When government policy encourages a flexible approach to the modes of program intervention, FBOs are able to establish "mutual interest" with other players towards improved health for the poorest people. However, this

59. Reich, "Reshaping the State from above, from within, from below," 1669.
60. AUSAID, "Helping Health Systems Deliver," 10–11.
61. Ibid.
62. AUSAID, "Helping Health Systems Deliver," 2.

approach requires the state to value the characteristics that define FBOs and the state needs to create space for people of faith to engage—without surrendering their *telos* and character.

An example of a state-centric initiative with significant influence on FBO practice has been the Millennium Development Goals (MDGs). The advantage of the MDG focus has been to give clarity and increase the potential for collaboration towards the outputs, outcomes, and impacts demanded by these ambitious goals. Saith identifies the positive value of the MDGs as the strength of good intentions, framed in the Millennium Declaration: the strength of solidarity and purpose—galvanizing the international community; and the benefits of instrumentality—providing a "template of targets for the bureaucratic mind."[63] However, this instrumental focus is a significant weakness. The MDGs are promoting a top-down, state-centric solution without sufficient resources being invested in stimulating grassroots response to achieve the outcomes, outputs, and impacts. A few years after they were agreed, the confident fervor of Jeffrey Sachs, a key architect of the MDGs and professor of economics at Harvard University, appears overoptimistic: "The MDGs depend critically on scaling up public health investment. As a matter of urgency developing world governments must present detailed investment plans that are sufficiently ambitious to meet the goals and the plans must be inserted into existing donor processes. Donor countries must keep their promises, which they can easily afford, to help improve health in developing world countries and ensure stability for the whole world."[64] In the light of the global economic downturn since 2008, it is unlikely that donors will be willing to fund a major increase in health care in the next few years. Even more significant are doubts regarding the developing world governments capacity to develop and implement "sufficiently ambitious" plans ensuring "stability for the whole world."

Another influential voice in the international development debate is Paul Collier, professor of economics at Oxford University. He is skeptical of the MDGs initiative but not skeptical about the power of the state. Rather, his recommendations expose a supreme confidence in the capacity of middle-to-low-income countries. Collier frames the issue of the

---

63. Saith, "From Universal Values to MDGs," 1167–68.
64. Sachs, "Health in the Developing World," 947.

poorest people through the lens of the state by arguing the MDGs unnecessarily include too many poor people.[65]

> The first critical lack of focus is that the MDGs track the progress of five billion of the six billion people on our planet. It is of course politically easier for the United Nations to include almost everyone. Plus the aid agencies prefer a wide definition of the development challenge because that justifies a near-global role for their staff. The price we pay is that our efforts are spread too thin and the strategies that are appropriate for the countries at the bottom get lost in the general babble. It is time to redefine the development problem as being about the countries of the bottom billion, the ones that are stuck in poverty."[66]

According to Collier, poor people living in economically developing countries—such as India, China, and Indonesia—should be excluded from the major aid focus because their countries are already prosperous, or at least on track to be so. Collier argues that every country was once poor and by avoiding the traps—the conflict trap, the natural resources trap, the trap of being landlocked with bad neighbors and the trap of bad governance in a small country—every country can develop. Karl Polanyi would be skeptical of Collier's confidence in the state as a key partner in resisting the commodification of the market. Polanyi was alert to the state's tendency towards unreliability—at times driving back markets but on other occasions being subservient to them.[67]

Collier does not adopt a skeptical position but, rather confidently, proposes a solution for the group of countries who are falling behind and often falling apart—and for whom the "bottom billion" have the misfortune to be citizens. Collier's recommends an interventionist approach to overcome the traps, strengthen the state, and encourage the market to drive economic growth. The weakness in Collier's argument is his simplistic starting point. He presumes that booming economic prosperity in places like India and Indonesia, with wealth often limited to the elite, will somehow translate into good health for the poor majority. Presumably, he concludes they are their government's problem and no one else's. Collier's recommendation to ignore the health of some of the poorest people merely on the grounds of their citizenship is not a faithful

65. Collier, *The Bottom Billion*, 3.
66. Ibid., 189.
67. Polanyi, *The Great Transformation*, 173–86.

response for FBOs. However, his analysis does highlight the significance of the state and some of the factors preventing the poorest people enjoying better health. These macro-issues are almost impossible for an FBO to influence but they significantly shape the context.

In summary, this section has shown a number of forces shaping the state in developing world countries. Despite its fragility, governments play a crucial role in improving the health of the poor. FBOs, NGOs, and foreign donors should not act in a way to undermine the state. However, the plight of the poorest people demands global attention and should not be left to governments who often lack the capacity and sometimes the inclination to respond. The MDG initiative is unlikely to achieve its targets but it is a useful means of focusing attention. FBOs should not ignore state-centric initiatives and can assist by ensuring process and relationship building is given priority over the instrumentality of many state-centric initiatives.

MARKET-CENTRIC RESPONSES

Following on from the assessment of state-centric solutions, this section reviews market-centric responses to the health of the poorest people. Markets continue to be promoted as the most efficient means of distributing health resources as long as they are left to function largely without institutional intervention in an unfettered global order. Although Polanyi's analysis shows this to be a flawed proposal, the provision of health care in developing countries is being increasingly shaped by market-centric presumptions.

Those who advocate most strongly for market-based approaches to improving the health of the poorest people have grave doubts about the ability of state-centric "solutions." William Easterly, professor of economics at New York University, presents a market-centric meta-narrative for improving the lives of the poor contrasting to the state-centric accounts offered by Sachs and Collier. Easterly argues for aid agencies to seek "home-grown, market-based development that will lift up both rich and poor" and for "western assistance for meeting the most desperate needs of the poor until home grown market-based development reaches them."[68] The aim of aid, Easterly says, should be to make individuals better off, not to transform societies or governments. He recommends the

68. Easterly, *The White Man's Burden*, 68.

ending of the existing official aid system and increasing a thousand-fold (at least) the number of individual, small experiments to stimulate the commercialization of society.

Easterly is critical of current market approaches in developing world health services—often with significant donor subsidies—such as competitive tendering, short-term renewable contracts, and performance measurement, which he argues, has led to a preoccupation with organizational survival and a willingness to deliver programs regardless of their utility. He recommends rewarding the "seekers" rather than the "planners" who innovate, stimulate, and replicate successful approaches free from the constrictions of state bureaucratic structures.

Easterly gives no account of how market forces—freed from donor and state control—will strengthen social relations. His faith in the market is undimmed. However, the expansion of the private health sector around the world has not been driven by the benefits it brings to the poorest people but by other factors such as the low quality of public provision and external pressure to liberalize the economy.[69] There has been some recognition in recent years of the importance of social agency but "constant repetition of commodification practices can only lead to further commodification no matter what the change in discourse and rhetoric."[70]

Health care for the poorest people requires funding from some source but it is unreasonable to presume the poorest people can meet the full cost. Therefore, it is not about whether subsidy is required but rather how it is spent. The market-based options currently advocated—user fees, private insurance, increased private involvement, and a decentralized role of the state[71]—are having limited success. The implementation of user-fees in Africa has generally not generated significant revenue and has made it more difficult for the poorest people to access health services.[72] There is some evidence indicating that indirect methods of payment help families pool the costs of accessing maternal health services and indirect methods are preferable to direct methods of payment.[73] Attempts to introduce German-style health insurance in low to middle income countries has

69. Mehrotra and Delamonica, "The Private Sector and Privatization in Social Services," 150ff.

70. Montiel, "Incompleteness of Post-Washington Consensus," 118.

71. Akin, "Financing Health Services in Developing Countries," 5–7.

72. Xu et al., "Understanding the Impact of Eliminating User Fees," 866.

73. Ensor and Ronoh, "Effective Financing of Maternal Health Services," 54–56.

been proposed as a means by which the state and market can coexist[74] but it is difficult to see the system working in poor countries with a history of poor governance. It is more likely to have success serving the middle to high-income groups rather than the poorest people in the developing world without massive donor subsidies.[75]

The harsh reality is that market-centric policies are not a panacea for the health of the poor. In fact, the cost of health care in a market-dominated society is pushing some people back into poverty. As noted in my field reflection from India the commodification of health care is particularly significant in South and East Asia resulting in billions of the poorest people being unable to afford and access appropriate health care. For example, more than 40 percent of the hospitalized patients in India borrow money or sell assets to cover expenses and in the process, 35 percent of these people fall below the poverty line.[76] The drive towards market-based solutions is being justified, by some, on the basis of the ineffectiveness and inefficiency of the state.

However, as Polanyi argued, the market and state are both inattentive to the impact of their actions on social relations. It is, therefore, in the interests of all members of society to find means of resisting market and state pressures. Public health practitioners generally appreciate the importance of social relations but appear unable to resist instrumental or market pressures.

THE MYTH OF THE "AUTONOMOUS RATIONAL INDIVIDUAL"

Before concluding this chapter, it is important to identify the understanding of "humans" underpinning many state-centric and market-centric solutions for the health of the poorest people. This book proposes an orientation for FBOs of "healthy persons" so, it is important to take a moment to describe alternative views. Central to Karl Polanyi's critique of the liberal market system, is his rejection of the utilitarian myth of *Homo oeconomicus*, "a creature motivated by self-interest, desirous only to maximize "utility" and guided by the rational calculation of

---

74. Barnighausen and Sauerborn, "One Hundred and Eighteen Years of the German Health Insurance System," 1560.
75. Janisch et al., "Demand Side Financing for Health Services," 1–23.
76. Varman and Vikas, "Rising Markets and Failing Health," 162.

opportunity costs."⁷⁷ This understanding of people underpins the liberal economic thesis in "that the foundational impulses of all economic activity emanate from rational, self-interested, economizing individuals."⁷⁸ This, as Polanyi shows, is a utopian view of humans, which results in an "artificial institutional assemblage against which society, understandably and rationally, reacts."⁷⁹

MacIntyre also critiques the increasing dominance of liberal individualism⁸⁰ and its understanding of person as individual moral agent: "freed from hierarchy and teleology, conceives of himself and is conceived of by moral philosophers, as sovereign in his moral authority."⁸¹ This limited anthropology of persons is particularly useful for the efficient functioning of the market-state. Persons become ends in themselves.⁸² Freed from the "burdens" of societal relations, shared *telos*, and the habits and practices of a faith-community, this "autonomous rational individual" is seen as having the capacity to solve his/her problems and plough her/his furrow. Excessive trust is placed in the capacity of science, human rights, and the inevitability of human development.⁸³ Reward comes from material success generated by the individual. It ends in a "survival of the fittest" society dominated by unfettered markets. It is not a healthy place for poor and vulnerable people.

In recent years there has been significant work within the discipline of economics questioning the traditional assumption of economic behavior as "autonomous," "rational" and "individual." Significant criticism has emerged of the restrictive character of traditional welfare economics with calls for greater appreciation of "wellbeing economics" and the role of relational goods in the promotion of wellbeing and welfare.⁸⁴ Atherton et al. identify an opportunity for a new stage in the relationship between economics and religion: "It has been a long journey from the seventeenth to the twenty-first century—from economics as the subject or servant of religion, via a reversal of that role by the later twentieth century, to the

77. Dale, *Karl Polanyi*, 91.
78. Ibid., 98.
79. Ibid., 72.
80. MacIntyre, *After Virtue*, 268.
81. Ibid., 62.
82. Rudman, *Concepts of Person and Christian Ethics*, 3.
83. Plant, "Does Faith Matter in Development?," 3.
84. Atherton, *Christianity and the New Social Order*, 66.

real opportunity now for religion to become an ally of economics in the pursuit of progressive change. And that alliance should also be regarded as an emblem or symbol of wider changes and possibilities, involving an increasing variety of disciplines and interests essential for the development of what Beccattini has called 'A new economy of wellbeing.'"

This move is to be welcomed and, as noted a number of times in this book, this is not the time for people of faith to become isolationist. If reciprocity and relationships become appreciated as having great significance in the reconstruction of the global economic system post the financial crisis of 2008, an appreciation of 'healthy persons' rather than "autonomous, rational, individuals' should be pre-eminent. As Rudman argues, the concept of persons is being given a position of "unparalleled regard in the competing value-systems of pluralistic societies."[85]

However, "unparalleled regard" often finds itself discarded in practice. My intention in highlighting the difference between an anthropology of persons as "autonomous rational individuals" as against "healthy persons" is to alert FBOs—and others—to the importance of appreciating that people are created in the image of God. People created to thrive as fundamentally relational beings with a common life that is more than individualistic "rational" choice. An appreciation of people as "healthy persons"—and the means of sustaining such an appreciation—will be developed throughout the remainder of this book.

---

85. Rudman, *Concepts of Person and Christian Ethics*, 3.

3

Health for the Poorest People beyond the State and the Market

MORE THAN 25 PERCENT of the world's population has no access to state or market health provision and rely on family and community plus their own ingenuity to stay healthy. Many other people are burdened with an ineffective state health service and/or unaffordable market provision. Therefore, it is essential to consider other key spheres of influence—apart from the market and the state—and their impact on the health of the poorest people. These forces include the community sphere, the Third Sector and Faith-Based Organizations (FBOs). In this chapter, I will also review the context of Salvation Army ministry with field reflections from Papua New Guinea and the Netherlands.

COMMUNITY-CENTRIC RESPONSES

Various terms can describe the "informal spheres" of human activity and relationships. Adalbert Evers, professor for comparative health and social policy at Justus Liebig University in Germany, defines "informal spheres" as "comprising families, informal social networks, and community building."[1] Other descriptors such as caste, tribe, and household can refer to the informal, non market-state sphere. I will use the generic descriptor "community" given its widespread currency among those seeking to improve the health of the poorest people. However, the word "community" often gives too great a sense of coherency to what are diverse, fluid,

---

1. Evers, "Part of the Welfare Mix," 160.

and fragmented forces of influence. I will highlight how this incoherency makes "the community" particularly vulnerable to co-option by the market-state.

Faced with a failing or disinterested state and an unaffordable market, many of the poorest people seek other means to improve their health. While the state and the market-centric approaches tend to focus on the individual citizen's rights and individual consumerism respectively, the community-centric approach emphasizes the importance of social relationships, social structures, and human capacity in responding to problems. Up until relatively recently, the family or household was the focus of attention for informal responses to health concerns. The importance of the household in the attainment of better health for the individuals has a strong public health evidence base. The 1978 Alma Ata Declaration called for a primary health care emphasis referring to the importance of "individuals and families in the community." In most low-income developing countries, the household is recognized as the most important producer of health. Decisions taken in the household have a significant impact on the health of the wider community.

However, in the 30 years since Alma Ata the emphasis has shifted away from the institution of family or household towards the term "community." The concept of "community" has flourished but it is difficult to define and lacks a specific institutional foundation within which to embed relations. Admittedly, accessing households and defining families is not straightforward—particularly in the chaotic neighborhoods where the poorest people often live—so community-centric responses prefer less defined concepts such as community, capacity building, and social cohesion.

Public health planners increasingly place expectations on the community's capacity to improve its own health.[2] Those promoting the capacity of communities to play a leading role in improving their own health often use a communitarian framework that contends society should articulate what is good. This contrasts with classic liberalism that holds each individual should be able to formulate the good on his or her own. Amitai Etzioni argues "community" can be defined with reasonable precision: "Community has two characteristics: first, a web of affect-laden relationships among a group of individuals, relationships that often crisscross and

---

2. Thomas et al., "The MESH Approach," 181–83.

reinforce one another (as opposed to one-on-one or chain-like individual relationship); and second, a measure of commitment to a set of shared values, norms, and meanings and a shared history and identity—in short, a particular culture."[3]

There are variations in the communitarian approach as to how society should articulate "the good." Asian communitarians promote the values of social order arguing that "in order to maintain social harmony, individual rights, and political liberties must be curtailed"[4] whereas responsive communitarians—often from western Europe or North America—hold that individuals who are well-integrated into society (rather than forced) are better able to reason and act in responsible ways than isolated individuals.[5] Critiques of community-centric responses raise examples of communitarian tolerance or even encouragement of oppression, authoritarianism, and conformity for the "greater good." According to Will Kymlicka, this oppression can entail the community prescribing roles of subordination, roles that limit people's individual potential and threaten their psychological well-being.[6]

In contrast to Asian communitarians who emphasize social order, African communitarians prioritize social relationships.[7] Family and tribe receive priority from this romantic community movement. In a corrective to liberal individualism, phrases such as "A person is a person through other persons" and "We are, therefore I am, and since I am, therefore we are"[8] capture the spirit of African communitarians as do terms such as "Ubuntu" and "community development." Criticism of African communitarianism arises over instances when individuality is subsumed by the collective and when relationships appear to override reason. For example, my wife, as a physician on the children's ward at Chikankata Hospital, Zambia in the late 1990s, was unable to stop a desperately sick child being taken off the ward by her father so his wife and the child could attend a funeral. The child subsequently died. The child's life was apparently less important than family obligations.

3. Etzioni, "Communitarianism," 224.
4. Ibid., 225.
5. Ibid.
6. (Kymlicka, 1993, 208–21) Source Etzioni, Ibid.
7. See www.africancommunitarians.com for examples of African communitarian writing.
8. Attributed to Dzobo on www.africancommunitarians.com.

An alliance in global health and community development has formed between responsive communitarians and individualistic liberalism. The western libertarians embrace the elevation of individualism in western societies in recent years and the rise of the "autonomous rational individual." This has resulted in a move away from a focus on concrete institutions such as "the family" towards the less defined concept of "community." The liberal market-state promises the "autonomous rational individual" full access to all possible rights but gives little attention to relationships or institutions such as family or household. This results in a collection of "autonomous rational individuals" being little more than an unconnected crowd rather than active participants in a relationally rich community.

However, western individualistic liberalism is at ease with the ill-defined notion of community for it no longer carries the specificity of institutions such as family, kith-and-kin or tribe. The western libertarians—who are more likely than African or Asian communitarians to be setting global health policy for NGOs and FBOs—have exported their suspicion of institutions (family, tribe, church) and, therefore, have a particular nervousness in working with faith-based institutions. The myth that secularism is a neutral position between belief and unbelief is widely accepted, despite its inherent absurdity.[9] The result is a tendency not to prioritize the role of institutions as means of sustaining community life nor a promotion of the practices and habits that sustain relationships.

Therefore, although Etzioni's definition of community—as webs of affect-laden relationships with a shared culture—is helpful, without the institutions of family, household or church around which to form and embed the webs of relationships, "the community" is a slippery and weightless construction. The combination of western libertarianism with non-western communitarianism leaves "the community" vulnerable to commodification and instrumentalization by the market-state and manipulation by powerful individuals within "the community."

This raises key questions for this book: What are the practices and habits needed to sustain the capacity of communities? If communities are a web of relationships, as Etzioni argues, what is the role of institutions (households, family, churches, etc) in enabling and sustaining the health of the poorest people? I return to these questions later.

9. Glenn, *The Ambiguous Embrace*, 20.

THE THIRD SECTOR AND THE RISK OF INSTITUTIONAL ISOMORPHISM

The practical theological reflection process used in this book enters into dialogue with other sources of knowledge to develop a deeper understanding of the situation.[10] This section turns to literature from organizational studies to gain insights into the context within which FBOs seek to improve the health of the poorest people. A framework proposed by Adalbert Evers, develops a space for the Third Sector as a part of a mixed welfare system—otherwise made up of the market, the state, and the informal sphere (comprising families, informal social networks, and community building).[11] In his recent work, Evers acknowledges the contribution of Karl Polanyi's analysis in the development of his account of Third Sector organizations. Evers appreciates the Third Sector as being "influenced simultaneously by different spheres that make up their social and historical context" and that the survival of the Third Sector "as something different, instead of adapting to the core values of state and market or regressing to informal settings and networks, cannot be taken for granted."[12]

Evers resists the tendency merely to perceive the Third Sector as another social service delivery agent operating from the same basis as either state or market providers. Rather, he construes the Third Sector as one dimension of the public space in civil societies, a tension field without clear boundaries where different rationales and discourses co-exist and intersect. It is an intermediate area rather than a clear-cut sector and therefore very exposed to tensions and influences coming from state institutions, the market economy, and the informal sphere of family and households.

Evers identifies "manifold interrelations" between the three main spheres—state, market, and the informal—on structural and historical levels. On the structural level, the dominant rationales are instrumental orientations (state), individual choice (market), and anonymity (informal sphere). Evers qualifies his construction of the anonymity of community by acknowledging that "norms and traditions of personal obligation and linkages are an important characteristic."[13] He notes

---

10. Swinton and Mowat, *Practical Theology and Qualitative Research*, 95–96.
11. Evers, "Part of the Welfare Mix," 160.
12. Evers and Laville, *The Third Sector in Europe*, 20.
13. Evers, "Part of the Welfare Mix," 163.

the dominance of commodification and commercialization in market economies and their tendency to restrict the room for the flourishing of public goods and services carried out by the state or Third Sector. He attributes a rise in financial prosperity as opening up new room for choices and anonymity for the individual while threatening to undermine community-based social relationships. It is in these circumstances that the Third Sector often experiences tensions as influences "compete, cross or have to be outbalanced."[14]

Evers calls for a greater awareness of the special nature of the Third Sector and for it to be viewed as different from business organizations. The complex scenario of "manifold interrelations" influencing state, market, and the informal sphere requires voluntary and non-profit organizations to be clear regarding their orientation. Evers notes that due to the dominance of economic considerations, the degree to which the strategies of the Third Sector are influenced by "ideological" factors are underestimated and too simplistically dismissed as "irrational." He also identifies the tendency of "church-based or bourgeois-linked charities" to turn into "quasi-market or state organizations by assimilating the respective rules, attitudes or discourses which dominate in the state bureaucracies or in the marketplace."[15]

Evers highlights how the dominating rationales in the state, market, and the informal sphere[16] are conditioned according to their historical context. Countries with a strong economic liberal tradition will prioritize the free choice of the consumer and tend to underplay people's roles and rights as citizens. Alternatively, nations with a socialist historical context focus have strong state-led concepts of progress and modernization dominated by universalist orientations. This leads to centrally planned and standardized service systems being viewed as the best way to guarantee equality.[17] In an era of globalization, nations are increasingly impacted by the consumerist discourse but even within that general orientation, Evers notes, there are national nuances attributable to historical causes.

14. Ibid.
15. Ibid., 165.
16. Ibid., 160.
17. Ibid., 164.

Evers identifies varying "orientations" for state, market, community, households and Third Sector spheres.[18] The dominating—and often fragmented and contradictory—orientations of state, market, and community cannot be ignored by a FBO as they can affect its character through the process of institutional isomorphism. Evers argues there is enough room for the Third Sector to operate despite a dominant state and/or market. He notes the Third Sector requires more than constitutional guarantees for a public space. Evers recommends a confident autonomous Third Sector that engages with market democracies to enable agreements and compromises by a process of exchanging and balancing viewpoints and interests. Evers proposes the cultivation of a civilized "culture of conflict" as means of engagement.

> This relationship between the public sector and the political majority on the one hand and non-profits and other organizations on the other can be referred to as conflictive co-operation. It does not exclude harsh conflicts, but instead it serves to limit them. Guaranteed rights for organizing concerns and a culture of conflict management in democratic countries has resulted in a tighter network of mutual contractual relationships between voluntary organizations and governments, balancing autonomy and integration. Hence, conflictive co-operation often seems to be the prevailing attitude beyond the alternatives of (self-) exclusion or symbiosis.[19]

CIVILIZED CULTURE OF CONFLICT

Using the conception of relations as a "civilized culture of conflict" Evers suggests four ways in which the Third Sector can relate to state, market, and communities. Firstly, the social and political role of Third Sector organizations is usually simply regarded in merely an economic role as alternative service provider. However, these organizations should not be simply understood—or see themselves—as economic providers of goods, services or practices. They are rooted in the cultural, social and ideological context and should be referred to as "a part of the whole tension field of the public space in a civil society."[20] Evers conceives a role for the Third

18. Ibid., 161.
19. Ibid., 167.
20. Ibid., 162.

Sector as a means of resisting the disembedding of social relations by the market-state as identified earlier by Polanyi. The degree to which the state and market allow space for the Third Sector varies. Evers notes that communist and fascist regimes tend to intentionally close down Third Sector space or incorporate their activities into the state. Equally the actions of a dominant neo-liberal market driven economy can also result in a closing down of non-market related space.

Secondly, Evers notes the potential for constructive Third Sector engagement not only with states and markets but also with the informal sphere—comprising families, informal social networks, and communities. Evers identifies the tensions that can arise in relations between the formal (market and state) and informal (communities, families, and households). Although seeming to base his analysis exclusively from western developed world perspectives, he identifies a broadening diversity of informal community cultures characterized by dynamics from "the traditional self reliant community" to a "defensive privatism of the modern small-scale household" contrasted with "more open forms of socializing" as people seek ways of maintaining anonymity with the need for personal exchange. This book accepts the complex dynamics contesting the space in the informal sphere and recommends attention to *telos* as an important response for FBOs.

Thirdly, Evers identifies an opportunity for the Third Sector to act as hybrids, intermeshing different resources and connecting different areas, rather than setting clear demarcation lines around a sector and mapping its size. Third Sector organizations are well placed to "act under multiple influence" from different areas and under conditions of parallel dependence. This can beneficially enable one organization to mediate or simply maneuver between different rationales and viewpoints in different sectors—a common characteristic of current Salvation Army practice[21]—but can also lead to tensions as the organization intermeshes

---

21. The diversity of Salvation Army social program is remarkable. In addition to health services, there are extensive programs supporting primary and senior schools, homeless hostels, elderly care institutions, children's homes, community care centers for children and elderly, domestic violence shelters, human trafficking responses, community development programs, etc. This leads to a culture of flexibility but also the risk of "mission creep." Charles Glenn's critique is insightful: "While few would fault the Army for being too charitable, it might be faulted for having an over inflated estimation of its own capacity to achieve sweeping social objectives" (Glenn, *The Ambiguous Embrace*, 216).

different tasks, roles, and rationales in contrast to the state or market who are "clearly dominated by a small number of specific rationales."[22] This is characterized by organizations relying simultaneously on market, state, and community-based resources; counterbalancing for-profit and non-profit activities and rationales; integrating paid work with voluntary commitment.

Fourthly, Evers identifies an opportunity for engagement for the Third Sector in a space between state, market, and community, which allows for "synergetic mixes of resources and rationales as opposed to substitution processes between different clear-cut sectors."[23] On a micro-level this enables Third Sector organization to facilitate the synergetic effects by more effective intersectoral combinations and networks of market, state, informal, and non-profit contributions. For example, the integrated continuum of care that is vitally important in primary health care in developing countries and requires synergy to maximize the use of limited resources.

This section has outlined Evers framework for envisioning a role for the Third Sector in a mixed welfare system. He recommends the various players accept the reality of "conflictive cooperation" as this will enable the Third Sector to sustain an independent space. I am in agreement with Evers's analysis as it applies to FBOs engaged in health ministry for the poorest people. For the Third Sector to play this intermediary role depends on their capacity to bridge the different rationales of state, market, and communities by constructively engaging with matters of concern while remaining faithful to their *telos*.

Evers acknowledges his indebtedness to Polanyi for this critique of the disembedding of social relations by market forces.[24] Evers uses Polanyi's concept of embeddedness to "highlight the complex totality of relations between public policy and initiatives in civil society."[25] This warning is helpful in describing and analyzing the context within which Salvation Army health ministry operates and differentiating between the spheres (market, state, informal). Evers argues for a differentiated space for the Third Sector and appreciates the teleological priorities for FBOs.

22. Evers, "Part of the Welfare Mix," 171.
23. Ibid., 160.
24. Evers and Laville, *The Third Sector in Europe*, 16–23.
25. Ibid., 22.

However, I have doubts about Evers proposal for establishing of common ground on the basis of "shared values and common sense."[26] I shall explore the issue of common ground later in this chapter.

FIELD REFLECTIONS

Evers highlights the danger for FBOs being domesticated by the state—a particular risk for The Salvation Army who, as will be seen in the following field reflections, is often dependent on government for funding its social services. This next section of the description and analysis of the context for contemporary Salvation Army health ministry outlines field reflections from Papua New Guinea and the Netherlands.

Papua New Guinea

Papua New Guinea (PNG), one of the most diverse countries in the world in terms of geography, biology, language, and culture, gained independence from Australia in 1975.[27] The young nation is challenged by mountainous terrain making transport links very difficult and costly and blighted by poor governance and corruption. There are more than 700 languages, over 1,000 dialects and many tribes, sub-tribes, clans, and sub-clans spread across its 20 provinces. PNG has abundant natural resources, although this has not led to economic prosperity for the majority of its people. In fact, the level of poverty has increased faster in recent years than in neighboring countries and PNG now ranks 148 out of 182 countries on the 2009 UNDP Human Development Index.[28]

An estimated 99 percent of the PNG population now identify themselves as Christians with at least 66 percent belonging to a denomination.[29] Church groups entered PNG in several waves since the late nineteenth century and PNG now has approximately 150 different missions, sects, and free churches.[30] The Salvation Army started in PNG in 1956—late in comparison with India (1882) and Zambia (1922). However, in terms

---

26. Evers, "Part of the Welfare Mix," 167.

27. During the Second World War, PNG was invaded by Japanese forces and, after being liberated by the Australians in 1945, became a United Nations trusteeship, administered by Australia.

28. United Nations Development Programme, "Human Development Report," 188.

29. Flaws, "The Church in Papua New Guinea," 4.

30. Hauck et al., "Ringing the Church Bell," v.

of current church member growth, PNG is one of the fastest growing Salvation Army territories in the world.[31]

Unlike India and Zambia, the church in PNG developed few hospitals but focused on developing primary health care programs. In partnership with the Australian colonial administration in PNG, the denominations opened health posts supported by seven church-run Community Health Workers training schools. The Salvation Army runs one of these training schools developing two-year trained Community Health Workers (CHW) who are employed by the churches to work in the rural areas (where 80 percent of Papua New Guineans live) at a health post. The CHWs work alone and are responsible for delivering a wide range of primary health care services including prevention, education, treatment, and care.

I visited several Salvation Army run health posts in 2008 and met a number of CHWs as well as the Salvation Army corps officers (congregational leaders) working at the adjoining corps. Although the health post and church share land, I noted variable levels of engagement. Where the health worker had a good relationship with the corps officer there was significant synergy released by integrating the clinical and pastoral work. However, there were tensions in some places which was not helped by an organizational divide in the management structure between the divisional commander (supervising corps officers) and the health services manager (supervising CHWs).

The relationship between the PNG state, the donors, and the churches is unusual. Although the PNG National Government has an impressive national health policy document—developed with significant support from the Government of Australia—it struggles with implementation.[32] The state is dependent on churches to deliver health services to at least half of the country's population. There is a widespread recognition that the churches play a central role in PNG society. In partnership with government, the churches co-manage some 40 percent of primary and secondary education facilities, run two of the country's six universities and are responsible for training many of the country's teachers and health workers.[33] The state has been praised for the quality of its relationship with the Church particularly in terms of service delivery and training of

---

31. Papua New Guinea has 11,316 adult members of The Salvation Army in comparison with 393 employees. The Salvation Army, *The Salvation Army Year Book 2010*.

32. Bolger et al., "Papua New Guinea's Health Sector," 10.

33. Hauck et al., "Ringing the Church Bell," 5.

community health workers.[34] The role of PNG church leaders has been shown to be effective in creating safe environments of care and support for those infected and for prevention of HIV.[35]

I noted significant skepticism among Papua New Guineans regarding the capacity of their government to deliver. People have more faith in the Church as a provider of social services. A history of chronic poor governance by the PNG state has forced western development agencies to have a more focused engagement with the Church. In turn, this has prompted churches to increase inter-church exchanges and cooperation and to give more serious consideration to their own internal management and governance.[36]

The Australian Government's development agency (AUSAID) recognized the value of engaging with the churches in PNG and funds not only the delivery costs of church health services but also church institutional capacity development. This includes training church leaders to equip them to better manage the delivery of social services to the PNG people. The Salvation Army is benefiting significantly from this funding for institutional capacity development. The PNG leadership of The Salvation Army are positive about the AUSAID funding. Unlike the normally restrictive funding from donor-states that can cause internal tensions and fragmentation, the AUSAID program was believed to have improved capacity and integration of Salvation Army ministry. I asked Salvation Army leaders about any negative influence resulting from taking comparatively large amounts of money from the state. I was told the PNG churches were alert to the dangers and were in a sufficient position of strength—comparative to the weakness of the state—to be able to resist demands from aid agency staff who "do not understand how churches function." Despite this optimism, there are some voices suggesting there is a risk of overestimating the potential of the PNG churches.[37]

This brief field reflection highlights the role of churches as more effective structures than the state for the delivery of health services. PNG is also noteworthy for a different form of institutional presence in communities with a move away from the typical large mission hospital model

---

34. Bolger et al., "Papua New Guinea's Health Sector," vii.
35. Benton, "Saints and Sinners," 315.
36. Hauck at al., "Ringing the Church Bell," 9.
37. Ibid., 20.

to small health posts and clinics closely linked to church congregations. This reflection also noted the influence of external donors upon the state and church—and apparently successful resistance by the church due to its clarity of purpose.

Netherlands

Charles Glenn, professor of educational leadership and development at Boston University, undertook a detailed study of the relationship between the Dutch state and the non-profit agencies. He argues that although many continue to claim a religious identity, there is considerable evidence that this has been "hollowed out" by decades of dependence upon the government as well as growing secularization in society.[38] NGOs who receive state subsidies are acquiescent to state demands and make their policies according to the government. Professionals care less about the identity of the organization than about professional codes. Glenn reports concern in The Netherlands about the "loss of the social middle" as a result of the incursions of bureaucracy on the one hand and markets on the other.[39] There has been a gradual handing-over of functions previously performed by families and the local community to civil society organizations. The increasing partnership between civil society organizations (including some FBOs) with the Dutch state "has led to institutionalization and professionalization of the function of human care of human beings."[40] Glenn argues there is more than efficiency and effectiveness at stake when governments turn to FBOs to act on their behalf: "There is an assumption that it is preferable to rely upon the churches to provide 'human care of human beings.' And perhaps more significantly . . . it is not a matter of open competition with new providers entering the 'market' all the time, but of long-established agreements with a few very large associations that occupy a near monopoly position in certain areas of public welfare."[41]

The Salvation Army in The Netherlands is one of these long-established large civil society organizations with significant public trust, receiving large government grants but a declining church membership. I visited the Netherlands on several occasions while researching this

38. Glenn, *The Ambiguous Embrace*, 139.
39. Ibid., 140.
40. Ibid.
41. Ibid., 131.

book and discussed these challenges with senior Salvation Army leaders. The most recently published statistics reveal that The Salvation Army in the Netherlands in 2009 had 4,871 employees compared to 5,836 adult members.[42] This is a significant shift—in 1989 there were 1,682 employees,[43] which increased to 2,227 in 1999. There has been a 20 percent decline in adult membership in the past decades from 7,310 in 1999 to 5,836 in 2009.[44]

In order to receive government funding The Salvation Army restructured in the 1980s with a clear organizational demarcation between the social services and the church. A degree of separation between church and social services has been demanded. I was told that in order to keep a faith influence in the social services, many of the most capable Salvation Army officers are appointed into the social service departments—resulting in a dearth of quality leadership in local corps (churches).

A senior leader of The Salvation Army in The Netherlands told me the church members feel they are the "little brother," overshadowed by the wealthy social services who increasingly employ professionally qualified staff with few links to the Salvationist worshipping community. Several other Salvation Army leaders said there was some jealousy among those engaged in corps work due to the large sums of money designated purely for social work and not available for evangelistic purposes. A number of Salvationist employees argued the problem was not with social services but was that corps were not "professional enough" and had been left behind. These disagreements resonate with Glenn's findings that as organizations become more oriented towards government, they become even more estranged from the religious rank-and-file with a resultant decline in the role of volunteering.[45]

Glenn argues The Salvation Army in the USA has done better than most American FBOs in resisting the pressures to conform to the state's agenda. Despite this, Glenn still identifies similar trends in the USA to those identified in The Netherlands:

---

42. These figures include both categories of adult members: soldiers and adherents. See The Salvation Army, *The Salvation Army Year Book 2010*, 185.

43. Idem., *The Salvation Army Year Book 1990*, 177.

44. Idem., *The Salvation Army Year Book 2000*, 162.

45. Glenn, *The Ambiguous Embrace*, 139.

The requirements of government contacting, coupled with the trend towards professionalization of care, have altered the character of some of the Salvation Army's programs, diluting the distinctive qualities that arguably have been key to its effectiveness in changing lives. The stated mission of the Army has remained relatively constant over time, yet its social services wing has gradually evolved from a grassroots, personal ministry into a large institutionalized operation increasingly detached from the religious life of its members. With only 83,000 adult members [in the USA], The Salvation Army has nearly 20,000 people on probation or parole assigned to them and provides help to 30 million (counting those who seek help repeatedly) a year.[46]

These two vignettes (PNG and Netherlands) identify pressures on The Salvation Army in both the "developed" and the "developing" world to comply with an agenda determined by the state (albeit in PNG a donor foreign state as well as the national government). The church in PNG appears to be able to manage the tensions but the loss of church membership in Netherlands is cause for concern. The result in the Netherlands has been some degree of dislocation between the FBO parts of Salvation Army ministry and the life of the worshipping community.

FAITH-BASED ORGANIZATIONS—LANDSCAPE

This chapter is describing and analyzing the context of Salvation Army health ministry for the poorest people. The preceding section of the chapter developed space for the Third Sector as part of a mixed welfare system otherwise made up of the market, the state, and the community sphere. As noted earlier, there are dangers for FBOs being lumped with civil society or the Third Sector. Therefore, it is important to describe and analyze the landscape within which FBOs operate.

For much of the twentieth century, the conventional wisdom was that religion was irrelevant to human development because, as nations "modernized," the influence of religion would inevitably decrease. Bretherton notes how modernization became identified with secularization and secularization was viewed as an inevitable outcome of the process of modernization such as industrialization, urbanization, specialization, and bureaucratization.[47] Wallace wrote in 1966, "The evolutionary future

---

46. Ibid., 213.
47. Bretherton, *Christianity and Contemporary Politics*, 11.

of religion is extinction . . . Belief in supernatural powers is doomed to die out, all over the world, as the result of the increasing adequacy and diffusion of scientific knowledge."[48] Such views became accepted leading to both religious and non-religious people internalizing the "secularization thesis" and it became a self-fulfilling prophecy.[49] Governments were often antipathetic to the social and political activities of FBOs, believing that secularism unites multi-faith societies and supports social stability in fragile nation-states.[50]

A number of factors have led to resurgence for matters of faith. Firstly, the demise of socialism and communism in the late 1980s and early 1990s (particularly since the collapse of the USSR) left a gap for the emergence of faith-based discourses in the absence of a credible social or communal-based narrative. For example, the rise of Hindu nationalism in India (with the rise of the *Bharatiya Janata Party* BJP) and the rise of Islam as a political force that generally went unappreciated by the West until 9/11. Since 11 September 2001, the political role of religion has been a subject of worldwide debate and engaging with people of faith in the developing world is no longer seen as something to be tolerated by western governments but an urgent priority. The "equality" prioritization in Western society did not allow governments to engage with Muslims only—all religions had to be engaged with on "equal" terms.[51]

Secondly, a factor resulting in significant growth in FBO activity, was increased government funding for FBOs, in the USA. The strict separation of state from church gave way to more accommodation and flexibility on the part of the state towards religion. Religion is an important part of American life and to the extent that a religious view is not privileged above others and no religious view is privileged over a nonreligious one, the state can work with FBOs for "the mutual enrichment of religion and American democracy."[52] This flexibility has developed partly as a result

---

48. Wallace, *Religion: An Anthropological View*, 265.

49. Bretherton, *Christianity and Contemporary Politics*, 11–12.

50. Clarke, "Faith Matters: Development and the Complex World of Faith-Based Organizations," 2.

51. Islamic NGOs operating south of the Sahara increased from 138 out of a total of 1,854 NGOs in 1980, to 891 out of 5,896 20 years later. Clarke argues many of the most dynamic Muslim NGOs nowadays combine proselytization with the provision of welfare services and a high standard of technical education. Ibid.

52. Bane et al., *Taking Faith Seriously*, xi.

of enlightenment secularism being understood as "comprehensive belief systems, which, like their religious counterparts, should not be privileged as the unifying basis of liberal democracy."[53] State-FBO partnerships are promoted by the state on the basis that FBOs offer flexible services, maintain pluralism, reinforce the norm of personal responsibility and limit the size of the welfare state.[54] The US Congress passed the Charitable Choice legislation in 1996 allowing religious organizations to apply for government grants as long as they did not discriminate on the basis of religion.

A third reason for increased interest in FBOs is the adoption of ambitious targets to tackle global poverty by the G8 group of world leaders. As the 2015 deadline approaches, it is understood that the Millennium Development Goals will not be attained without partnering with people of faith. Engaging with FBOs is not a straightforward task for most western governments. Many state employees are faith-illiterate and view FBO partnerships as "counter-development or culturally exotic to a secular and technocratic worldview."[55] Admittedly, their task is not easy. There are a bewildering complexity and diversity of FBOs and NGOs—some with blatantly self-serving agendas.[56] It is a complex challenge for the state and other agencies to determine whom to engage with and upon what terms.

FBOs should view with some caution the newfound interest from government bodies for engaging with matters of faith. The state tends to view FBO partnerships as a means towards the end of better health for the poorest people. This is unlikely to be "Damascus Road" conversion of the nation-state towards a faithful orientation for health ministry but rather a pragmatic, instrumental move on the basis of their geo-political priorities. Many FBOs are encouraged—even excited—by this new willingness to partner after years of struggling to secure funding. However, the impact of partnerships on FBOs needs careful consideration.

Luke Bretherton, from a British perspective, identifies "multiple modernities" affecting the shape of state-faith relations, each with their respective relationship to religious belief and practices overlapping and interacting within the same shared, predominately urban, spaces.[57]

---

53. Ibid., 7.
54. Smith and Sosin, "The Varieties of Faith-Related Agencies," 651.
55. Clarke, "Faith Matters," 32–3.
56. de Gruchy, "Of Agency, Assets and Appreciation," 29.
57. Bretherton, *Christianity and Contemporary Politics*, p15.

Although these multiple modernities are not present in every place around the world, they are influential in shaping Western donor policy and, in this way, have an impact.

This section has described some of the features of the landscape within which FBOs operate. It has noted the following significant forces shaping the FBO landscape: the decline of the secularization thesis, the demise of socialism, and communism, the rise of militant Islam and Hinduism, the increased US funding to FBOs, and the instrumental needs of the state to improve the health of the poorest and its need to partner with people of faith.

FAITH BASED ORGANIZATION—TYPOLOGIES

Describing and analyzing the landscape confronting FBOs as they seek to improve the health of the poorest people is essential but it is also important to understand the variations of faith within FBOs themselves. FBOs do not all share the same faith, are not all orientated by the same *telos*, they do not speak one common language, nor do they exhibit the same characteristics. This section will engage with the academic literature to identify types of FBOs and locate Salvation Army health ministry within a typology.

The academic literature on typologies of "developing" world FBOs is limited. The African Religious Health Assets Programme (ARHAP) undertook an extensive literature review and mapping exercise in sub-Saharan Africa.[58] One of their conclusions was to opt for the term "religious entity" (RE) in preference to FBO. This is justified on the basis that FBO fails to capture the reality of religious formations in Africa. The term FBO, they argue, fails to reflect "that many of the most religious responses do not have fixed organizational status."[59] In a more recent work, Jill Olivier describes in detail the myriad ways FBOs have been defined over the last ten years in the context of HIV/AIDS in sub-Saharan Africa.[60] Olivier argues little has been gained from typologies developed in Africa and notes a lack of information regarding the impact of external funding upon REs in Africa.[61]

58. Olivier et al., "Working in a Bounded Field of Unknowing," 16.
59. Haddad et al., "The Potential and Perils of Partnership," 3.
60. Olivier, "In Search of Common Ground," 89.
61. Ibid., 88–108.

The experience in western countries of state-FBO partnerships may be more instructive. There has been a large amount of research into FBOs in an American context.[62] Ronald Sider and Heidi Unruh's meta-analysis identifies commonalities between FBO typologies. Firstly, the concept of religious integration is common—the notion that "religion is not an independent attribute but a dynamic that is incorporated into the organization in a variety of ways and intensities."[63] The second commonality is an appreciation that whether an organization is faith-based cannot be simply answered yes or no. The faith nature of organizations is multidimensional, requiring a range of types. Sider and Unruh developed a typology to assess "meaningful and measurable ranges of religious integration" by focusing on "observable and explicit phenomena" within an established set of organizational dynamics and religious elements to construct a model of the ways that religion is manifested in FBOs.[64] The typology has a dual focus—both organizational attributes such as resources, governance and staffing as well as the nature of religious practices in program methodologies.

Sider and Unruh's typology is based on eight religious practice characteristics and four religious program characteristics. From these characteristics a six-fold typology is constructed. The types of FBOs identified are faith-permeated, faith-centered, faith-affiliated, faith background, faith-secular partnership, and secular.[65] Based on my field reflections and experience, Salvation Army health programs tend towards two of Sider and Unruh's typologies—faith-centered and faith-affiliated.

> "*Faith-centered* organizations were founded for a religious purpose, remain strongly connected with the religious community through funding sources and affiliation and require the governing board and most staff to share the organization's faith commitments. Faith-centered programs incorporate explicitly religious messages and activities but are designed so that participants can readily opt out of these activities and still expect the benefits of the program's services."

---

62. Jeavons, *When the Bottom Line Is Faithfulness*, Smith and Sosin, "The Varieties of Faith-Related Agencies."

63. Sider and Unruh, "Typology of Religious Characteristics of Social Service and Educational Organizations and Programs," 116.

64. Ibid.

65. Ibid., 120.

> "*Faith-affiliated* organizations retain some of the influence of their religious founders (such as in their mission statement) but do not require staff to affirm religious beliefs or practices, with the possible exception of some board and executive leaders. Although faith-affiliated programs incorporate little or no explicitly religious content, they may affirm faith in a general way and make spiritual resources available to participants. Faith-affiliated programs may have the intent of conveying a religious message through nonverbal acts of compassion and care."[66]

However, if orientated by a *telos* of "healthy persons," Salvation Army health ministry may be more typified as "faith permeated." "In *faith-permeated* organizations the connection with religious faith is evident at all levels of mission, staffing, governance, and support. Faith-permeated programs extensively integrate explicitly religious content. The religious dimension is believed to be essential to the program's effectiveness and therefore participation in religious elements is often required."[67]

This typology focuses on the character of the FBO—as evidenced in their characteristics—as being most significant in determining the typology of the FBO. Sider and Unruh's typology does not, however, evaluate the various characteristics in terms of "faithfulness." Yet, the neo-institutional theory upon which the typology is constructed is sensitive to the forces that cause the character of FBOs to change. The process of change, institutional isomorphism, is particularly important in describing and analyzing the terms upon which "common ground" is established between FBOs and the other spheres influencing the health of the poorest people.

THE SEARCH FOR "COMMON GROUND"

Finding "common ground" with other organizations involved in health work in particular location is becoming a priority for The Salvation Army health ministry in developing countries. Western government donors are increasingly demanding partnerships as a precondition to funding. There is a push towards more funds being allocated in-country rather than being approved in the capital cities such as Washington, London or Oslo. The donors are placing similar requirements on recipient governments

---

66. Ibid.
67. Ibid., 119.

through the Sector Wide Approaches (SWAPs) initiative.[68] The result of this pressure from the western donor establishment is requiring FBOs to make "common ground" with an increasing number of partners. However, as previously argued, the dangers of isomorphism are significant.

FBOs cannot and should not avoid partnerships. The process of isomorphism does not need to be inevitable. Smith and Sosin argue that if FBOs make conscious choices, they can shape their organizational character. This process of shaping is dependent on the degree to which faith is coupled with the allocation of resources, the choice of partnerships, and the dominant sources of authority. The less the FBO is coupled to the faith community, the more the FBO will be coupled to secular society. "The tighter the coupling to religion, the more an agency's social organization reflects the demands of that religion."[69] Therefore, the choices made by FBOs are of critical importance. Identifying the frameworks upon which FBOs make those choices is foundational to understanding the extent of coupling. Therefore, this section will describe and analyze three proposals for establishing "common ground" between people of faith and the world in which they live.

Dignity and rights framework

Smith and Sosen identified a "relative uniformity" among FBOs in certain underlying assumptions. They identified a common dignity and rights framework as foundational among FBO's conception of the principles underpinning their engagement with people who do not share their faith commitment. This is achieved by respecting their rights and preserving their dignity. For example, the researchers interviewed Salvation Army leaders in Seattle and Chicago who said no client was required to participate in religious programming because the leaders believed this to be "demeaning."[70] By adopting this framework, the researchers concluded, FBOs justify their place in public life on the basis that religion serves the individual and the wider community by providing positive experiences that enhance life. FBO's reliance on the dignity-and-rights framework enables them to distinguish themselves from secular providers but also

---

68. AUSAID, "Helping Health Systems Deliver," 10–11.
69. Smith and Sosin, "The Varieties of Faith-Related Agencies," 656.
70. Ibid., 660.

keeps them consistent with many demands of secular culture, such as avoiding discrimination on the basis of religion.

Smith and Sosin suggest the dignity and rights framework offers a productive "common ground" for engagement of FBOs and the wider society.[71] However, it could also be argued that FBOs are merely adapting to normative isomorphic pressures from the prevailing culture which pressurizes the FBOs into accepting a secularized dignity and rights framework—based on the concept of the "autonomous rational individual" rather than the concept of "healthy persons."

African experiences seeking "common ground"

Jill Olivier reflects on the experience of faith-based groups seeking common ground in the African context—particularly impacted in the past two decades by HIV/AIDS and the subsequent flood of donor dollars. As a doctoral student, Olivier worked with the African Religious Health Assets Programme, who describe themselves as an intentional formation of "a community of enquiry at the intersection between religion and public health" and defined "common ground" as "shared values, shared goals, or a shared language."[72]

Olivier identifies some of the challenges in seeking "common ground." "While there may be more frequent conversation between religious and secular institutions and individuals, communication, and partnership continues to be hampered by misunderstandings, frustrations or a 'communication gap.'"[73] Olivier notes that the key to establishing and sustaining common ground is relationships. "The real successes of ARHAP have been developed over time, through countless conversations, arguments, and discussions and in the development of relationships."[74] She also appreciates that it takes a long time and requires commitment of the community of inquiry to a long-term process[75] and notes: "Common ground and common language is not developed by glossing over arguments or

---

71. Ibid., 665.
72. Olivier, "In Search of Common Ground," 66.
73. Ibid., 6.
74. Ibid., 175.
75. Ibid., 176.

rapid definitional work, but rather in appreciating difference, in constantly interrogating difference through dialectical argument."[76]

To this point I am in full agreement with Olivier. However, Olivier goes on to argue that common ground can be created by "bringing out potential commonalities underlying the conflicting disciplinary and theory-based insights so that these can be reconciled and ultimately integrated."[77] Olivier proposes "common ground" on the basis of the shared vision of "social justice" as a "boundary concept that draws diverse language together."[78] This proposal for "social justice" as shared vision is problematic. As Alasdair MacIntyre has extensively argued, justice should not be decoupled from the practices and habits that sustain it.[79] Without shared practices and habits, "social justice" becomes a hollow construct, a blank sheet upon which to project a variety of perceptions of justice.

I suggest "shared vision" is an unrealistic expectation for the diversity of people and groups seeking to improve the health of the poorest people. A more realistic position is to establish "mutual interest" and a willingness to work across boundaries for the common good in a civilized culture of conflict, as proposed by Adalbert Evers. A "mutual interest" position does not require people to accept a shared *telos* but opens up the potential for working together despite alternative *telos*. Common ground will not be easily established with shared *telos* or a "dignity and rights" framework but, rather, on the basis of "mutual interest." People with a diversity of backgrounds and ambitions can discover "mutual interest"—as for example, with the health of the poorest people—despite different *telos*.

This "mutual interest" approach is not without significant tensions. It requires a significant degree of humility and dwelling in places of tension. However, this is a faithful place for FBOs to inhabit. The church needs to live not only with tensions but "deliberately and actively cultivate" them.[80] At the same time, the state must be willing to open up (or, at least, not close down) spaces for people of different faiths and values to work together despite alternate *telos* driven by a variety of faith convictions.

---

76. Ibid.
77. Ibid., 66.
78. Ibid., 173.
79. MacIntyre, *Whose Justice?*
80. Hunter, *To Change the World*, 279.

Interrelated roles and practices as the basis for "common ground"

A multi-disciplinary enquiry under the auspices of Harvard University has articulated the quest for "common ground" on the basis on "mutual interest." They propose an appreciation of the interrelated roles and functions of FBOs and the secular liberal state as the basis of "common ground." The editors of *Taking Faith Seriously* argue: "Because so much of religion's contributions are good for democracy and because these contributions are anchored in faithful religious practices, we propose that creative initiatives to strengthen the intrinsic religious practices of faith communities will also serve the instrumental aims of helping to strengthen pluralist civil society and participatory democracy."[81]

This is a constructive starting point that seeks to find areas of mutual interest between the secular liberal state and the faith community by allowing different ends (*telos*) to be attributed to the same action by different groups. The FBO is enabled to rely on "faithful religious practices" with the understanding that the results are acceptable because they strengthen the instrumental aims of the state.

Bane et al. propose a "common ground" based on six interrelated roles or functions for FBOs working within a liberal democracy: fostering expression; forming identities; creating social bonds; shaping moral discourse; enabling participation; and providing social services.[82] They deliberately leave the provision of social services to the last point believing that too much focus is placed on it to the exclusion of other critically important roles and functions. Bane et al. identify several legitimate concerns such as FBO service capacity, a lack of a culture of accountability; an absence of sound empirical research; concern regarding proselytizing vulnerable clients and discriminatory employment practices. They argue it is very important for FBOs to have greater certainty when making partnerships with other organizations and be explicit regarding what they can—and cannot—bring to the table.

Ronald Thiemann rejects the secularist demand that FBOs distinguish between the "religious" and "nonreligious" elements as an impossibility due to communities of faith developing out of rich, dense, and constantly changing traditions with complicated relationships between the faith community and the host society contributing to fundamental

---

81. Bane et al., *Taking Faith Seriously*, 311.
82. Ibid., 8.

changes within each. He argues: "Despite the evident complexity of religious organizations, social scientists continue to search for a means by which the "distinctively religious" dimension of complicated social relationships can be identified and isolated."[83]

The unrealistic proposition by dogmatic secularists that FBOs stay away from health services or at least have "different" rather than "common" ground[84] is unreasonable. Thus, "common ground" can be forged by FBOs and secular liberal states not by agreeing the *telos* but rather by appreciating the value of the role or function from the differing standpoint of the polity, secular organizations or religious organizations. Such arrangements should permit a variety of interpretive analysis of narrative, identity, and mission as well as a diversity of functional analysis over resources, actions, and outcomes. This apparently slippery position can be sustained if the role and function of FBOs as an instrumental contribution to the pluralist democracy is respected as being anchored in the intrinsic commitments of religious faith. As Bane et al conclude: "Many religious practices involve such intrinsic commitments as trust in, and obedience to God, openness to the sacred and service to the neighbor. Thus we are not merely making the instrumental claim that religion fosters community and good character for the sake of the polity; we propose that many of the same practices that benefit democracy are anchored in faithfulness as practiced in many religious traditions."[85]

However, sustaining such a position requires FBOs to maintain confidence and consistency in their inherently public character by living out the beliefs upon which the FBO is established. This conclusion resonates with a study of faith-based agencies in five Western democracies that concluded the greatest threat to FBO autonomy came less from regulation by government than from what they call "changing norms of religious schools and agencies."[86] In other words, the greatest threat to the character of FBOs comes from within.

In summary, this section argues the terms upon which FBOs establish partnerships is significant. A number of frameworks for the building of "common ground" were presented: a common vision of rights; social

---

83. Thiemann, "Lutheran Social Ministry in Transition," 178.
84. de Kadt, "On Keeping God out of Development," 1.
85. Bane et al., *Taking Faith Seriously*, 303.
86. Monsma and Soper, *The Challenge of Pluralism*, 108.

justice; and contributing to the common good. The latter is recommended as it enables FBOs to maintain a faithful *telos* sustained by distinctive habits and practices while also serving the instrumental aims of the nation-state and wider society. Therefore, a vital task for leaders of FBOs is to ensure their organization is clear about its *telos*, intentional in sustaining a distinctive character, habits, and practices while being alert to the threat of institutional isomorphism. Admittedly, this is a place of tension-dwelling but this is typical of the faithful presence required of FBOs engaged in improving the health of the poorest people. This proposal is developed in Chapter 5 through the process of theological reflection.

HEALTHY INSTITUTIONS?

The previous section recommended FBOs should be attentive to the *terms* upon which "common ground" is established in the quest to improve the health of the poorest people. This section will consider the *means* by which the distinctive character, habits, and practices of people of faith can be sustained in the cause of improving the health of the poorest people. This book seeks to recover an appreciation for the contribution of *institutions*—such as congregations, clinics, and hospitals[87]—for the task of improving the health of the poorest people.

Institutions lost credibility in the twentieth century—particularly in western societies—as the structures of modernity came under scrutiny from post-modern thought. Institutions such as church, hospital, school, government, and corporations became viewed with suspicion as their capacity to abuse power was better appreciated. One response to the loss of trust in institutions has been a rise in the popularity of community-centric solutions. These, allegedly, are "free" from the institutional power abuses. As has been argued earlier, this is a naïve conception of the sources of power in communities—whose power arrangements can also damage relationships and fail to improve the health of the poorest people. I am not proposing a return to the institutions of modernity but neither is it endorsing any romantic illusions arising from post-modernity. Power

---

87. I am using the term clinic/hospital to cover a variety of faith-based health institutions. While I argue for the value of an institutional presence in this thesis, health institutions should be as small as possible. Pressure from developing world Christians to develop large hospitals is, I will argue, a product of commercialization rather than evidence of faithfulness. Therefore, priority is given to clinics rather than hospitals but for simplicity I combine the two with the term clinic/hospital.

is understood as a given of social life. All people—Christians and non-Christians—wield power in relationships, institutions, and organizations of which they are a part. As Hunter explains: "The question is how we will use whatever power we have ... Wherever power is exercised, it needs to be orientated by a self-giving compassion for the needs of others—within and outside of the church."[88]

This final section of Chapter 3 describes and analyses the current contribution as well as the potential of clinics, hospitals, and congregations. It will be argued that the power of institutions is not uncontrollable and can be faithfully orientated. Institutions can play a key role as building blocks of a more complex space that FBOs should promote against what Bretherton calls "the totalizing, monopolistic thrust of the modern market and state that seek to instrumentalize and commodify persons and the relationships between them."[89] Without such institutions, people struggle to have the opportunity to dialogue, free from government or commercial imperatives. Such spaces are essential if people are to have the space and time to listen to each other and develop mutual trust.[90]

Clinic and hospital-based ministry

For the past 20 years, FBOs have moved away from promoting and funding hospitals and clinics in preference for community-based health programs. Western donors are reluctant to fund institutionally based health services believing their money is better invested in "the community." This move towards de-institutionalized health care is a major departure from the expansion strategy adopted by the western Church up until the 1960s. A negative view of health institutions was (and continues to be) influenced by the perilous state of many church mission hospitals. Most large faith-based hospitals in the developing world are economically unsustainable and a number of denominations face the same problems.[91] In 2001, an independent, interdenominational investigation into Christian mission hospitals in developing countries identified six issues threatening their future—lack of vision and leadership; staffing; community relationships;

---

88. Hunter, *To Change the World*, 247.
89. Bretherton, "A Postsecular Politics?," 19.
90. Ibid.
91. Crespo, "The Future of Christian Hospitals in Developing Countries," 3–7.

finance; cultural conflicts; technology.[92] A brief reflection on the development of health institutions will provide an important context for contemporary initiatives.

In the nineteenth and early twentieth century, the growth of the Church in many developing countries was linked to the development of education and health care.[93] The church embarked on an extensive expansion of institutions such as schools, clinics, and hospitals—usually in collaboration with the colonial rulers. These institutions were promoted as a means of developing the colonies and its people and required significant personal sacrifice by western missionaries. The health and education institutions generally proved popular with the local people. However, almost all western clinicians rejected indigenous healing practices and relied upon the western bio-medical model of healthcare.[94]

The roots of the rise of Protestant medical missions in developing countries reside in eighteenth century Wesleyan revivalism with a concern for the eternal salvation of the individual rather than a priority for the transformation of society.[95] Seeing poor health in local communities, the first missionaries concluded "preaching without healing was a most inadequate way of interpreting the Gospel."[96] Neither Hinduism nor Islam had developed institutional health services for the poor as an expression of their faith and the dedication of the missionaries impressed the local people.[97] Tensions arose with the missionaries' desire to proselytize. Most missionaries were sensitive to the tension but pressure came from denominational leaders who viewed evangelism as eternally essential.[98] Most clinicians were similarly convicted and the necessity of long periods of recuperation in hospitals for patients offered opportunities for relationship building and faith sharing.

Since the 1960s there has been a waning of interest in Christian hospitals. Currently, most mission hospitals are run by national staff and are struggling to survive due to a lack of resources and, in some cases,

---

92. Ibid., 3.
93. Grundmann, *Sent to Heal!*, 30–37.
94. Evans, *The Healing Church*, 16.
95. Garlick, *The Wholeness of Man*, 133.
96. Ibid., 48.
97. Ibid.
98. Evans, *The Healing Church*, 16–17.

management skills. In other instances, denominations have withdrawn completely and handed the institutions back to the government. A variety of reasons have been given to justify western donor withdrawal from mission hospitals in developing countries. Abigail Rian Evans identifies the following:

> "The recent paradigm shift in the Two Thirds World is moving health care delivery from the hospital-based medical missionary movement model towards an integrated health-and-community based model, empowering people to be responsible for their own health. The reasons for this shift are (1) the exorbitant cost of establishing and sustaining health institutions; (2) alternative sources of health care provided by government and private organizations in many countries; (3) the difficulty by a number of countries in managing large medical institutions that exceed local competency levels and specialties; and (4) the shift in North American missiology from building institutions to empowering and enabling people in preventative health care based on a holistic, communitarian view of health."[99]

Charles Glenn provides an insightful theological perspective on decline of imperialism and its impact on missiology. He argues one outcome of Protestant theological reflection in the later half of the twentieth century was a valuing of the secular for its own sake: "The more the secular sphere was seen as rich in signs of grace, the less urgent and even credible was it to seek to bring a revelation-based understanding to bear upon social problems. Religious people should just roll up their sleeves and join in the world's work—especially the struggle for racial and economic justice—without any pretensions to special insights or agendas. A 'servant Church' should not seek to impose itself upon the world."[100]

Glenn links the rise in Protestantism of an appreciation of the secular with the anti-imperialist spirit engulfing the post-1945 world. This resulted in the abandonment of foreign missionary evangelistic efforts. In preference, western churches began to restrict their activities to simply offering practical care, such as health ministry, with a reluctance to acknowledge any faith distinctive. In retrospect, Glenn argues: "It is clear that the provision of assistance unrelated to evangelism was simply

99. Ibid., 17.
100. Glenn, *The Ambiguous Embrace*, 243.

a transition to complete abandonment of the missionary enterprise."[101] Glenn notes the almost complete withdrawal of western protestant missionaries from the developing world.

Glenn's conclusions resonate with my reflections. I fear that apart from a regular flow of short-term, western "mission tourists," who generally gain more from the visit than their gracious developing world hosts, the developing church is being left alone to navigate a future orientation for faith-based health ministry. Some support is offered by western-based FBOs with loose links to denominations but these FBOs have increasingly close ties to large government donor grants. This brings with it the threat of institutional isomorphism.

Patricia Wittberg's research into Catholic religious, Protestant deaconesses and women's missionary societies notes a common decline—or complete loss—in the denominations' links with Christian social institutions in many parts of the world. Using a neo-institutional framework of analysis, Wittberg identifies the process impacting both institution and denomination: "To the extent the differentiation processes are leaching religion from schools, hospitals, social service agencies, and the like, some degree of isomorphic pressure is probably responsible. And the privatization of religion and personal belief may well be a response of church members—especially virtuoso members of religious orders or mission societies—to the attenuation of a meaningful religious culture in these organizations, as well as to the lack of an operant connecting tie between sponsor and institution."[102]

The changing relationships that resulted from reduced links between the institution and denomination are significant for this book. Wittberg identifies how the weakened or severed institutional ties have affected the institution and denomination's internal and external identity, changed the focus of activities, impacted the professional development of the nuns and sisters—and the loss of power has reduced the women's ability to influence their denomination and wider society. Organizations rarely notice how much their identity has changed and the process of reformation is "a time-consuming, contentious, and dangerous process" resulting in many institutions and denominations avoiding the issue until a severe crisis leaves them with no alternative but to address the topic.

---

101. Ibid.
102. Wittberg, *From Piety to Professionalism*, 16.

Catholic hospitals in the USA[103] have constantly evolved starting from the religious order providing the service, before supervising others to provide it and finally to controlling the boards of hospitals who administer the provision of services.[104]

This analysis is similar to the experience of Christian hospitals in developing countries. Initially, health services were provided by missionary doctors and nurses who, then, trained local people to work under their supervision. This arrangement lasted for most of the twentieth century. However, in recent years the number of western missionary doctors and nurses has declined. At about the same time there was a reduction in financial support for institutional health care from western donors. The situation is further complicated by insufficient numbers of developing world Christians with appropriate skills willing to work in under-resourced hospitals resulting in the recruitment of people with an inadequate understanding of the distinctive characteristics of faith-based health ministry. The influence of the denomination on the institution is now often limited to controlling the boards of hospitals while clinicians prioritize professional standards in the delivery of medical services.

What is the way forward? Developing world church leaders still see the need for church hospitals to serve the poorest people in their communities but are struggling to find the necessary resources. While accepting there is no reason to sustain institutions merely because they are cherished trophies of a long-gone era, the costs of closure need to be carefully considered. Health care institutions can have a constructive role if they contribute to an integrated health system that gives priority to community-based health care working with local congregations. Hospitals and clinics are usually among the most sophisticated institutions in an area inhabited by poor and vulnerable people. Montiel noted the importance of institutions as one of the flexible elements of social processes capable of dealing with changing circumstances. Nevertheless,

---

103. By the mid-1920s, Catholic health care in the USA became a particularly dominant force with 60 percent of all hospital beds in Catholic hospitals—compared to 12 percent in European hospitals. This situation remained unchanged until the 1970s. Almost all US Catholic hospitals were founded and owned by religious orders and not by the dioceses themselves. Despite significant reduction in recent years, Catholic hospitals in the USA continue to serve more than 89.1 million inpatients and outpatients annually. The 623 Catholic hospitals represent over 11 percent of the nation's total community hospitals and over 13 percent of all U.S. community hospital admissions.

104. Wittberg, *From Piety to Professionalism*, 59–72.

he argues, institutions are in no position to guarantee any specific outcome at all, unless they are considered as a tool that the situated agents in context might employ.[105] In concord with Montiel's argument, I propose health institutions function as a hub for the governance, negotiation, coordination, and regulation of community-based health care as well as building trust with the population as an effective link in a continuum of health care from home to hospital and back.

This is the conception of the health institution in the community that this book wishes to promote—a health institution as a resource upon which all community members can be supported and influenced through a "dense web of relationships" and in doing so they contribute to the sustainability and quality of the health facility.[106] I use the term "clinic-hospital" in referring to this conception of a health institution. Few large, multi-specialty, mission hospitals—built in the 1950s and 1960s by missionaries with grandiose plans—will survive in the competitive twenty-first century market-driven health context. This book is not promoting a return to that vision of faith-based health institution. Rather, small, focused, quality clinic-hospitals that are orientated towards faith-based health initiatives as close to the family as possible, sustained, and resourced by the worshipping community, will be recommended in Chapter 6.

The crisis facing mission hospitals should be a significant issue of concern for denominational leaders around the world. The historical roots of church congregations and mission institutions in developing countries are deeply entwined. The Salvation Army—and this applies also to other denominations—will be significantly weakened in the next 30 years unless attention is paid to recovering a faithful role for institutions in twenty-first century mission. The current situation is unfaithful and unsustainable. Seeking to relive past glories cannot be the basis for a faithful future. A reformation process towards clinic-hospitals is required.

Congregation-based health ministry

This chapter seeks to describe and analyze options for the health of the poorest people beyond those offered by the state and market—particularly responses by people of faith. The previous section promoted

---

105. Montiel, "Incompleteness of Post-Washington Consensus," 120.
106. Faguet and Ali, "Making Reform Work," 211.

clinic-hospitals as an institutional resource against the often destructive behavior of the market-state. However, more important than clinic-hospitals is the contribution of congregations who work together, with people of other faiths, for the common good. Congregations should not function—or be perceived—merely as groups of people who regularly worship God together for their own benefit. Rather congregations, as an outcome of their creed and worship, seek the common good for all people, without discrimination. Jeavons argues this is a key question in defining the contribution of the church to society: "Do these organizations and the activities they undertake, primarily serve their own members or a larger public?"[107]

There is a long tradition of congregations as public benefit organizations[108] and in the face of faltering state health provision, marketplace medicine, increased longevity, the spiraling cost of health and the increase in lifestyle illnesses,[109] the focus of public health strategists has shifted from institutionally-based services to developing capacity in individuals, households, and communities—and increasingly faith communities. The Church plays a key role in many parts of the "developing" world and new forms of congregation-based health care are attracting interest from western donors. This mirrors the donor government's domestic strategies—particularly in the USA.[110] The bio-medical model of health care is proving too costly, the technologization of health care is compounding the issue and congregation-based health-care is being proposed. Evans promotes the church functioning "as a health institution and a healing community by basing its ministry on a broader definition of health as wholeness, sickness as brokenness and healers as those persons who assist us towards health. The church is the corporate expression of the individual Christian's calling to a healing ministry. It can contribute to our personal movement towards health as well as furnish part of a concrete health care system."[111]

The poorest people in developing countries struggle to access market-state health care. One of the few institutions likely to be accessible to

---

107. Jeavons, *When the Bottom Line Is Faithfulness*, 41.
108. Ibid., 45.
109. Such as heart disease, obesity, type 2 diabetes, etc
110. Evans, *The Healing Church*, x.
111. de Gruchy, "Of Agency, Assets and Appreciation," 21.

the rural villager as well as the slum dweller is the local congregation. It is particularly well placed to support primary health care programs including education, prevention, and care initiatives. Treatment programs can also be considered but these are more costly and will usually require the participation of a health professional. This is an area of partnership between congregations and clinic-hospitals. Therefore, the expansion of congregation-based health services should be encouraged by FBOs but a number of concerns should be noted.

Firstly, the tendency for congregations to want to "do something" about the plight of "the poor" rather than seek identification and engagement with the shared task of developing "healthy persons." Steve de Gruchy rightly questioned the "do something" approach: "In making this fundamental assumption of being 'not able to do,' are we not simply mirroring the power dynamics that lie at the heart of the experience of poverty and hence reinforcing the very problem we think we are solving?"[112] Such an unreflective activist approach results in the agency of poorer people—their ability to act independently—being under recognized and rarely nurtured by the church. This is particularly a risk when delivering treatment services where it is easy to slip into an instrumental—viewing "the poor" as a means to an end—rather than relational understanding of people. Thus, it is critically important that congregation-based health ministries (and other FBO health services) affirm, enhance and appreciate the agency and identity of poor people themselves in the task of improving their own health. This approach embraces two important theological principles: the poorest people appreciated as both made in the image of God *and* called to be actors in the drama of creation and salvation itself.

A second area of concern is the trend by FBOs—encouraged by state funding agencies—to prefer community-based health programs rather than congregation-based initiatives. FBOs undertaking a community-based program tend to invite the church to join the discussion but only as one voice among many. People of faith—particularly in poorer communities—are being encouraged by global health and development community to accept "responsibility" to empower ordinary people, by all means possible. However, the faith resources, habits, and practices of the worshipping community are rarely utilized. As argued previously, the weightless concept of community is more acceptable than a theological

112. Ibid., 24.

rich appreciation of congregation. Improving the health of the poorest people is being orientated by an aspiration towards the "autonomous rational individual" rather than an eschatological *telos* of "healthy persons." Therefore, the church is viewed as one community asset among many; a valuable resource for improving the health of the poorest people but not given any priority as the body of Christ in the world.

A third area of concern relates to the isomorphic impact of faith-based health ministries upon the life of the congregation. The emphasis placed on congregational-based health ministry—based on the US parish nursing experience—is proving effective in several developing countries and acknowledged as a critical link in providing access to health care. Congregation-based health programs in Zambia and India as well as mosque-based services in Kenya and Uganda received positive reviews from USAID.[113] However, tensions can arise in the relationship between the congregation, the community and the faith-based institution. Tensions can arise between clinic-hospitals (who tend to use paid workers) and congregations (who tend to depend on volunteers).

The final section of Chapter 3 has reflected on the challenges and opportunities for faith-based clinic-hospitals and congregations. It has concluded that clinic-hospitals can play an important and often underestimated, role and benefit from close links with congregations. Congregations have capacity and calling to be more than "mutual benefit organizations"[114] and can work for the common good when attention is given to sustaining faithful presence and resisting isomorphic pressures.

SUMMARY

This chapter has undertaken a cultural and contextual analysis of the spheres of influence beyond the market-state that affect the health of the poorest people. While accepting contextual differences between different parts of the world, this book seeks an international orientation for Salvation Army health ministry enabling a faithful engagement with a number of common spheres (market, state, informal) in order that the poorest people in the world enjoy better health.

A critique of community-centric responses was developed. The slipperiness and weightlessness of a de-institutionalized conception of

---

113. Chand and Pattison, "Faith Based Models," 10–12.
114. Jeavons, *When the Bottom Line Is Faithfulness*, 45.

community were noted. Evers' framework of a mixed welfare system offered a distinctive Third Sector that engages, challenges, and keeps the market-state under close attention. Field reflections from Papua New Guinea and the Netherlands enriched the analysis with insights from contemporary practice. This book resists any collapsing of FBOs into the Third Sector and argues it is impossible to agree a common *telos* for all the spheres operant in the mixed welfare system.

The chapter explored the forces shaping the landscape and the types of FBOs engaging in health services. The process of institutional isomorphism, it was argued, is not inevitable but FBOs should pay close attention to their own frameworks of decision-making as these are unlikely to be the same as those of the state, market or wider society. Therefore, common ground should be attempted not on the basis of *telos* but rather through a commitment to discovering *mutual interest* and creating space that appreciates the differing standpoints of the polity, secular organizations or religious organizations. Such tension dwelling enables a diversity of interpretive and functional responses for the common good.

The chapter concluded with a review of the contribution of health institutions and congregations to the task of improving the health of the poorest people. I have argued that closing them down and abdicating to market and state provision will not faithfully resolve the crisis facing many mission hospitals in developing countries. Faithfulness demands a refounding process. The purpose of the refounding is to reorientate clinic-hospitals so they can nurture the health and agency of the poorest people. This is also a role of service for the wider church community within an impoverished neighborhood. The poorest people require the support of institutions, such as the congregation and the clinic-hospital, to resist pressure from forces of instrumentalization and commodification from the market-state as well as self-seeking manipulation from powerful individuals.

The next chapter continues with Stage Two of Swinton and Mowat's model of practical theological reflection to develop an understanding of the cultural and contextual challenges facing Salvation Army health ministry.

4

Health for the Poorest People: Salvation Army Responses

THIS CHAPTER DOES NOT present a history of Salvation Army health ministry. As this chapter will show, the majority of academic research on The Salvation Army has, to date, used the tools of the historian. In contrast, I am attempting to develop a practical theology and I hope this will become the preferred mode of enquiry for Salvationist scholars in the future.

Swinton and Mowat note the importance of "practices" in the work of a practical theologian. Practices such as preaching, prayer, hospitality, caring for the sick, or enabling community development initiatives contain their own "particular theological meanings, social, and theological histories, implicit and explicit norms and moral expectations. The ways in which we practice and the forms of practice in which we participate are therefore filled with deep meaning, purpose and direction."[1] There is, relative to other denominations, a limited pool of academic literature on Salvation Army theology and practice. There is an extremely limited amount specifically focusing on health ministry. Therefore, I have included in my analysis of Salvation Army practice the broader area of Salvation Army social services—of which health ministry is one expression.

I have chosen to reflect on Salvation Army practice through an engagement with three writers who have been particularly influential in the development of Salvation Army theology and practice—John Wesley,

---

1. Swinton and Mowat, *Practical Theology and Qualitative Research*, 19.

William Booth, and Philip Needham. Firstly, John Wesley's theology was, and remains, influential in The Salvation Army. What follows is not a comprehensive assessment of Wesley's health theology but rather a brief sketch so to set the scene for a fuller analysis of William Booth's work. William and Catherine Booth, the founders of The Salvation Army, were members of the Methodist Church. William Booth was a Methodist minister before resigning. Wesley's appreciation of the contribution of medicine in the congregational life of the church is informative in understanding The Salvation Army context.

Having briefly sketched Wesley's theology of health, I reflect on William Booth's influential book, *In Darkest England and the Way Out*, published in 1890 in dialogue with other Salvation Army literature from that era. Finally, I reflect on the implications for Salvation Army practice in the writings of Philip Needham, an influential Salvation Army officer whose thinking has shaped contemporary Salvation Army health ministry. The chapter concludes by identifying particular areas of Salvation Army practice requiring further reflection in the light of Christian soteriology, missiology, and eschatology.

JOHN WESLEY ON HEALTH AND MEDICINE

Medicine is, from Wesley's perspective, a "good" as long as health care practices do not distract humans from the proper union with God. Wesley is "best understood as one fundamentally committed to a therapeutic view of Christian life"[2] who reflected on the Christian experience of salvation as the recovery of holiness of body and soul. The physical—as well as the spiritual—health of the poorest people was a priority for Wesley.

Wesley lived at the dawn of the Enlightenment and was influenced by the spirit of his age as he witnessed rapid advances in technology and science. However, he appreciated the limitations of science or, as it was called, natural philosophy. His understanding of healing was rooted in the love and grace of God, which was manifested, not only in the progress of knowledge in the modern world, but also in supernatural healings, which transcended natural philosophy and science.[3] Despite this theological priority, Wesley's interest in natural philosophy and the dominance of the

---

2. Maddox, *Responsible Grace*, 23.
3. Webster, "Health of Soul and Health of Body," 218.

mechanical metaphor in the early days of the industrial revolution affects his theology significantly. He develops a structured, almost mechanical, staged soteriology. Felleman notes: "The normative religious experience, the "life of God in the soul of man" as John Wesley sometimes referred to it, was available to all who repented of their sins, were saved by faith, born again, and pursued inward and outward holiness. The developmental steps in this order of salvation—conversion, justification, regeneration, and sanctification—are discussed, defended, and defined in countless sermons, hymns, poems, and treatises. If these steps were diligently followed, Wesley claimed they normally led to a feeling of happiness in the spiritually mature."[4]

Wesley also has a mechanistic understanding of medicine and health with an almost Gnostic understanding of the body describing it as an "animal machine" with a literal understanding of the effects of the Fall.[5] He suggests, when Adam and Eve ate the fruit in the Garden of Eden, the fruit released into the body "particles that began to adhere to the inner coats of the finer vessels." Strictures within the vessels laid "a foundation for numberless disorders in all parts of the machine" and signaled the inevitable process of death.[6] Despite Wesley's mechanistic understanding, he did conceive of a symbiotic relationship between body and spirit (soul). He does not devalue the body to a "thing" and the well-working body is fundamental to Wesley's concept of health. When and where the body is impaired, the total person is diminished.[7]

Randy Maddox provides a helpful assessment of Wesley's theological and relational anthropology[8] and concludes that "allowing for some dualistic influences ... Wesley's two-dimensional anthropology (body-soul) did not degenerate into a strong metaphysical or ethical dualism. His basic anthropological convictions sought to emulate the holism of biblical teaching."[9] However, Maddox admits Wesley's "valuation of bodiliness was not as positive and his conception of the interrelationship of

---

4. Felleman, "A Necessary Relationship," 140.
5. Wesley, *The Works of John Wesley*, 219.
6. Ott, "John Wesley on Health as Wholeness," 47.
7. Ibid., 55.
8. Maddox, *Responsible Grace*, 68–73.
9. Ibid., 72.

body and soul was not as integral and dynamic, as present theologians might desire."[10]

Health, for Wesley, is a fundamental good insofar as it enables Christians to participate in God's work of redeeming the world. Wesley's understanding of health was shaped by the concept of a well-working body. It is easy, with the benefits of hindsight, to critique Wesley's scientific assumptions and methods[11] but Wesley drew on the best medical knowledge of the day. However, what is important to note is Wesley's orientation—his *telos*. Wesley focused on eternal health for all in Christ now and in eternity through the integration of body and soul. Wesley taught that Christian love arose from faith and was "a reaction to the experience of God's love and forgiveness. Real Christians have an inward demonstration, evidence, and conviction of their redemption made possible by faith."[12] Methodists, influenced by Wesley's teaching, promoted the idea that God's healing presence was available for all individuals in society. Thus, their embracing of supernatural healing had a social and religious impact during the Enlightenment. However, all the advances of science and medicine were gifts of God's grace and should not be disparaged or discarded in the pursuit of health and wholeness.[13]

Wesley's interest in medical science was subservient to his theology of God. If the medical facts supported his theology he was willing to work with it—but he questioned the science if it clashed with the theology. He promoted the use of natural medicine and spiritual prayers in combination as a means of achieving improved health. There were times when Wesley prioritized prayer over medical practice but, more often, he advocated the use of medical intervention as well as prayer—an integrated approach to the healing of both body and soul. Wesley's interest in new medical techniques was not primarily in new technology but rather in its use to improve the health of the poorest people.[14] He did not encourage his followers to visit the sick only as a means

---

10. Ibid.

11. For example, In *Primitive Physic*, Wesley reports an experiment sealing a cat in a sealed box with a lighted candle and noting the cat's death coincided with the extinguishing of the candle. This was before science had identified oxygen but Wesley concluded there was some life giving force in air.

12. Felleman, "A Necessary Relationship," 158.

13. Webster, "Health of Soul and Health of Body," 226.

14. Schwab, "'This Curious and Important Subject,'" 202.

of pastoral care, but proposed a treatment plan for various illnesses to complement the pastoral ministry.[15] Wesley wished to ensure "the widest possible access to safe, inexpensive, and effective ways of getting and keeping well."[16] He had a concern for the health of the poorest people and was skeptical of the practice of contemporary medicine. He suspected physicians preferred "exotics" over simple remedies.[17] In this respect, Wesley's critique is still relevant given the ravages of market-driven medicine in contemporary practice.

Central to Wesley's *telos* was not simply the health of the body but rather the recovery of holiness in all aspects of life. Hauerwas acknowledges the importance of Wesley's contribution in recovering the centrality of holiness as integral to the Christian life, in that, central to Wesley's theology was "the singleness of intentions, the constancy of character, that makes our behavior consistent with a life totally devoted to God."[18] Wesley emphasizes sanctification and importance of evidence of predictable and manifest change of character.[19] Wesley's conception of Christians as pilgrim people undertaking an arduous but fulfilling journey reveals the teleological dimensions of Wesley's redemptive understanding. For Wesley (and Hauerwas) the journey must result in positive change, but this change is not as a result of our abilities but "the sovereignty of God's grace over our sinfulness."[20]

Hauerwas believes Wesley's emphasis on constancy of character and evidence of sanctification is still relevant today as we now live in a world "just beginning to be born in Wesley's time—a world that no longer assumes that a religious, or in particular, a Christian account of life is necessary for decent and upright living. What difference, if any, it makes to be a Christian becomes even more pressing in such a world."[21] Hauerwas appreciates Wesley's inherently teleological account but has some concern with the priority given to the stages of "perfection" in sanctification. Hauerwas argues Wesley was "unable to find the appropriate

---

15. Webster, "'Health of Soul and Health of Body,'" 216.
16. Schwab, "'This Curious and Important Subject,'" 202.
17. Ibid., 180.
18. Hauerwas, *Sanctify Them in the Truth*, 131.
19. Ibid., 123ff.
20. Ibid., 124.
21. Ibid., 125.

means to suggest how our being on a journey also requires results in the particular kind of singleness characteristic of Christians."[22] Hauerwas notes MacIntyre's point about the difficulty of characterizing constancy is almost exactly parallel to Wesley's stress on perfection.[23] Perfection needs a "reference to the wholeness of human life" but that is not easy. Wesley was aware of this risk and tried to overcome it by, yet again, adopting a mechanistic solution. According to Hauerwas, Wesley makes his teleological framework primary and makes "justification but one step along the road. As a result he fell into unfortunate language of 'stages' in an attempt to characterize perfection . . . The problem with his scheme, of course, is that it is too neat, for Wesley was acutely aware that our lives can hardly be laid out with such exactness. Stages overlap and we regress."[24]

Where Wesley, Hauerwas, and I concur is that a concept of "perfection" is necessary in describing the *telos* of any adequate account of the Christian life. "Moreover, it places that emphasis rightly—for the teleology is not one of moral decisions or justifications, but of the self."[25] Hauerwas is right to wish Wesley had found a less controversial word than perfection. Perfection unfortunately conveys "too much of a sense of accomplishment rather than the necessity of continued growth that was at the heart of Wesley's account of sanctification."[26] Despite Wesley's language of perfection, Hauerwas argues it is unnecessary to contemporize it with terms such as "maturing" or "wholeness." Rather, he prioritizes the task of re-imagining how to characterize perfection. For Hauerwas as for Wesley, the character and evidence of perfection in the Christian life is most important. "The demand to locate and characterize lives of perfection is fundamentally a communal task. For the journey Christians undertake is the journey of a people. The growth of individual lives, which certainly is also a journey, is intelligible only within the movement we call church."[27]

Key points can be drawn from this discussion on Wesley's relationship with medicine. Firstly, Wesley appreciated a theological anthropology

22. Ibid., 126.
23. Ibid.
24. Ibid., 127–28.
25. Ibid., 142.
26. Ibid., 124.
27. Ibid., 141.

of persons as united body-soul. He understood the purpose of medicine to be, therefore, getting and keeping the body well so it can serve the greater purposes of God—as against being an instrument, commodity or servant of another power. Secondly, there is immediacy to Wesley's eschatological *telos* allowing for recovery in the here-and-now. Wesley promoted the *telos* of health as the recovery of complete holiness in every aspect of life. This is helpful for this book seeking a *telos* for health ministry characterized by a constant desire for continual improvement and the attainment of excellence to the extent that fulfills the greater soteriological purposes of God.

WILLIAM BOOTH AND IN DARKEST ENGLAND AND THE WAY OUT

William and Catherine Booth founded The Salvation Army in 1865 after William had spent 15 years as a Methodist New Connexion preacher. William said of himself: "I worshipped everything that bore the name of Methodist. To me there was one God and John Wesley was his prophet . . . I cared little then or afterwards for ecclesiastical creeds or forms. What I wanted to see was an organization with the salvation of the world as its supreme ambition and object."[28]

By 1890, William Booth's grand design for transforming the world was not through preaching individual salvation and holiness alone. Informed by the experience of working in the East End of London and his Wesleyan heritage, William Booth appreciated that people required total transformation, including physical, social relationships with family, friends, society, the work place, and the nation. Indeed, Booth conceived of The Salvation Army playing a key role in the total transformation of the whole world for God. Roger Green, the leading contemporary Salvationist historian, highlights the importance of understanding William Booth's motivations. He was not ministering to the poor in order to create a more stable society. Rather, "Booth was primarily an evangelist and a revivalist, pressing the hope that spiritual regeneration would manifest itself in social stability."[29] This conclusion is foundational to this book. William Booth's *telos* was theological, not sociological.

---

28. Booth-Tucker, *The Life of Catherine Booth*, 52.
29. Green, *The Life and Ministry of William Booth*, 109.

Booth's Problem Analysis

Booth wrote *In Darkest England and the Way Out* against a background of social unrest and growing political concern.[30] In 1889, London Dockers had been on strike and Charles Booth—no relation—published the first volume of *The Life and Labour of the People of London*, an inquiry into the condition of the capital's poor.[31] Charles Booth provided a scientific analysis of the problem but offered few solutions. William Booth, ever the pragmatist, decided it was time to set out his solution. The structure of *In Darkest England* has similarities with a basic practical theology framework. Booth identifies the issue, describes, and analyses the problems; reviews alternative options and then proposes his grand plan for revised practice. However, despite my assertion that Booth's *telos* was theological, there are few explicit references to theological resources shaping his arguments. I will return to this deficiency after briefly describing the structure of the book.

In the first chapters of *In Darkest England*, William Booth identifies the problem of extreme poverty in England—particularly in the large cities and goes on to describe and analyze the plight of a group of people he terms "the submerged tenth"[32] who are ignored by the wealthier parts of English society. He taps into the fascination of Victorians with "Darkest Africa"[33] and uses it as a metaphor, arguing that the situation in the East End slums is just as bad as life in the Congo.[34] Booth seeks to shake the complacency of "Christian" England, comprising people who, in his assessment, were "self righteous and detached."[35]

Booth analyses and describes the problems of homelessness, work, alcohol, prostitution, crime, and education. He provides quantitative data and uses qualitative case studies of people helped by The Salvation Army to give a personal dimension to the problems facing the poorest people. Booth is critical of other solutions. He has little confidence in the capacity

---

30. Hattersley, *Blood and Fire*, 353.
31. Ibid., 344.
32. Booth, *In Darkest England*, 16–23.
33. Henry Morton Stanley captured the public imagination in his writings about journeying across Africa in *Through The Dark Continent*.
34. Booth, *In Darkest England*, 9–15.
35. Ibid., 84.

of the poorest people to solve their own problems.[36] Booth dismisses the effectiveness of the state as an organ of redemption[37] and is critical of other solutions such as prisons,[38] charity,[39] emigration, trade unionism, and thrift.[40]

Booth is alert to the disembedding of social relations—as described by Karl Polanyi half a century later. Booth gives the example of the typical "good neighborliness" in small communities where neighbors know each other. Tools are shared and loans are made not on the basis of the competitive market but embedded in the social relations of the community. Booth identifies value in the principle that "the honor of the family is a security upon which a man may safely advance a small sum." However, Booth laments: "In the large city, all this kindly helpfulness disappears and with it go all those small acts of service which are, as it were, the buffers which save men from being crushed to death against the iron walls of circumstances. We must try to replace them in some way or other if we are to get back, not to the Garden of Eden, but to the ordinary conditions of life, as they exist in a healthy, small community."[41]

Booth's solutions are not isolationist. He did not refuse to work with the state or the market capitalists of his day such as Cecil John Rhodes[42] but engaged with them in the confident expectation that he could change their practice. Booth set out seven "essentials to success"[43] including changing the character and circumstances of the poorest people through a sufficiently large, permanent, immediately practical scheme that would not harm its intended beneficiaries or "seriously interfere with the interests of another."[44] These "essentials to success" highlight the difficulty in describing the book as a piece of practical theology.

In contrast with his other writings, Booth reduces the theological content of his argument in this book. Perhaps in seeking to appeal to a

---

36. Ibid., 44. "Some men seem to have lost even the very faculty of self-help. There is an immense lack of common sense and of vital energy on the part of the multitudes."

37. Ibid., 67.

38. Ibid., 73.

39. Ibid., 72.

40. Ibid., 78.

41. Ibid., 217.

42. Hattersley, *Blood and Fire*, 427–28.

43. Booth, *In Darkest England*, 85–89.

44. Ibid., 87.

wider audience to secure financial support for his scheme, Booth fails to clearly articulate the role of faith in the transformation of the character of the individual. While he identifies "character change" as the first of the seven "essentials to success," he does not specifically link it a Christological soteriology. At one point Booth appears to drift towards an individualistic salvation of humanity by human scheme when he muses: "Is it too much to hope that in God's world God's children may be able to do something if they set to work with a will?"[45]

Although *In Darkest England* adopts the structure of a reflective process, it is not an adequate practical theology as it lacks the explicit theological content evident in William and Catherine Booth's writings. Thus, in describing and analyzing Salvation Army culture and context in the light of practical theology, I include other early Salvation Army texts for theological insights.

Booth's Grand Plan

In *In Darkest England*, William Booth claimed to have a scheme that would be as significant in changing the world as the invention of the railway.[46] With echoes of Wesley's mechanical understanding of the body and disease, Booth proposes a mechanistic solution for the ills of society and suggests parallels with the industrial revolution: "What we have to do in the philanthropic sphere is to find some thing analogous to the engineers' parallel bars. This discovery I think I have made and hence have I written this book."[47] Included in Booth's proposals were a number of innovative environmentally friendly recycling initiatives[48] that he argues would re-balance "the societal machine by human action."[49]

Booth's plan was, in effect, a scheme for the re-embedding of social relations against the forces of the unregulated market in Victorian England. Booth summarizes his intentions thus: "The Scheme I have to offer consists in the formation of these people into self-helping and self-sustaining communities, each being a kind of co-operative society,

---

45. Ibid., 88.
46. Ibid., 89.
47. Ibid.
48. The Salvation Army formed Household Salvage Brigades to collect and recycle bones, sardine cans, packing cases, ropes, waste paper. I visited similar programs continuing today in Mumbai and Kolkata in India.
49. Booth, *In Darkest England*, 114–23.

or patriarchal family, governed, and disciplined on the principles which have already proved so effective in the Salvation Army."[50]

Central to the process of building "self-helping and self-sustaining communities" was the role of institutions. Booth proposes three primary institutions: The City Colony, The Farm Colony, and The Overseas Colony. Working out of these colonies could be a number of institutions all seeking to develop the capacity of individuals, families, and the wider community. Booth's scheme is highly dependent on institutions. In *Darkest England* he dedicates a chapter to the development of institutional responses such as industrial schools, children's refuges, asylums for moral lunatics, workshops for unemployed, rescue homes for women, hostels for drunkards, social agencies (labor bureau); the poor man's bank, the poor man's lawyer, and model suburban villages.[51] Booth argued the institutions that sustain the upper and middle classes as well as the poor in rural areas and villages should be available for the poorest people in the cities. Many of Booth's institutions appear to be counter-movements against the actions of the market-state in Victorian England.

Booth places great faith in the value of work, discipline, and organization[52] and appears comfortable in using market practices in achieving the ends of the *Darkest England* scheme. Booth is quick to differentiate the scheme from "charity" insisting it is "work for the workless."[53] Booth had high expectations for the "submerged tenth" but insisted they must be compelled to participate[54] and if they refuse, they should be permanently secluded from the world.[55]

The one problem facing the "submerged tenth" in Victorian England for which Booth does not propose an institutional response was their physical health. Instead of proposing the establishment of hospitals or clinics, Booth proposes a primary health mobile clinic staffed by nurses. He muses:

> I have been thinking, that if a little Van, drawn by a pony, could be fitted up with what is ordinarily required by the sick and dying

---

50. Ibid., 91.
51. Ibid., 90–93.
52. Ibid., 90.
53. Ibid.
54. Ibid., 206.
55. Ibid., 204.

and trot around these abodes of desolation with a couple of nurses trained for the business, it might be of immense service without being very costly. They could have a few simple instruments so as to draw a tooth or lance an abscess and what was absolutely requisite for simple surgical operations. A little oil stove for hot water to prepare a poultice, or a hot foment, or a soap wash, and a number of other necessities for nursing could be carried with ease.[56]

He was initially resistant to his eldest son, Bramwell's, recommendation to open up institutional medical work in India in 1893. John Coutts reports in his history, "The old man took some persuading. Might not the care of sick bodies divert attention from the salvation of perishing souls? But at last he agreed."[57]

By 1907, Bramwell was less enthusiastic about hospitals and doctors. He wrote to his father: "It is evident that the Hospital and Dispensary work is going to be a torture to us owing to the doctors; their wants and fads and prejudices and professional conceits and their consciousness they evidently have in the background all the time, that they can go away and earn three or four times the money we pay them and all that sort of thing, making them exceedingly difficult to deal with . . . Whatever we do, we must have some proper regulations for them. Now we have absolutely nothing."[58]

It appears from this brief insight into the practice of health ministry in The Salvation Army that institutional responses have been an ongoing challenge. These same issues continued to challenge Salvation Army health ministry during the next 110 years: the poor people's need for quality, affordable hospital services; the potential benefits for poor people from community based health care; a concern that health ministry diverts Salvationists from the evangelical task; the complexity of running health institutions and sustaining a faithful ministry in the face of pressures from commercialism and professionalism.

William Booth is attentive to the importance of informal institutions and seeks to strengthen their capacity. I give two examples from *In Darkest England*—the family and the trade unions. Booth notes the actions of state and market in disrupting family life by offering emigration only to productive individuals—husbands were separated from wives

---

56. Ibid., 178.
57. Coutts, *The Salvationists*, 142.
58. Booth, *Personal Communication with William Booth*.

and children. Booth promised The Salvation Army's emigration scheme to his Overseas Colonies would ensure all members of the family stayed together.[59] Secondly, the unions: On several occasions when explaining his plans to create work Booth is concerned not to upset the unions and reassures them that it is not his intention to undercut the wages paid to people in employment.[60]

Booth is respectful but skeptical of the capacity of the state to solve the problems of the poorest people. He hopes, in due course, the state will take over some of the activities[61] but he fears the actions of the market will undermine the state.[62] Booth does not lack confidence or vision for the role of The Salvation Army even suggesting, in the absence of the state, setting up a Salvation Army Court of Arbitration to "mother" society by resolving disputes.[63] He accepts people will object to the scope of his scheme and argue many of his proposals should be the responsibility of the state but Booth questions its ability to deliver. Booth estimates his scheme will cost £1 million and argues this is not much in comparison with the Afghan war, which was costing £21 million.[64] In matters colonial, Booth is far too confident in the benefits of imperialism. He does not appear to doubt the state's role abroad despite his critique of its ineffectiveness at home.

Booth's scheme was faith-based but he included few references to other denominations. Booth's Salvation Army was highly critical of the religious establishment of the day and defined itself as a "movement" not a church. Salvationists understood themselves to be participating in a movement of the Spirit to transform the world for God. Salvationists believed God raised up the movement distinct from the ineffective Church. Their understanding of this task of saving the world was based on a post-millennial theology with The Salvation Army playing a central role. However, I contend, the resonance of Booth's scheme beyond the ranks of faithful Salvationists was due to The Salvation Army's credibility in resisting the ravages of the market-state upon the poorest people.

59. Idem., *In Darkest England*, 152.
60. Ibid., 108.
61. Ibid., 215.
62. Ibid., 216.
63. Ibid., 226.
64. Ibid., 251.

THE FAITH FOUNDATIONS OF BOOTH'S SCHEME

In Darkest England cannot be regarded as a piece of practical theology as it lacks explicit theological reflection. However, reading *In Darkest England* in light of Booth's other writings reveal his theological priorities and the contribution of theology to Salvation Army practice. This section will reflect on four issues: personhood, missiology, *telos,* and relations with the world.

Booth's understanding of personhood

William Booth's conception of the anthropology of persons—as well as his missiology and eschatology—transformed The Salvation Army from a successful, but small, expression of militant holiness into a global Christian mission to the unconverted, poor, and oppressed. GM Trevelyan, the English social historian, wrote in 1942: "The Salvation Army regarded social work and care for the material conditions of the poor and the outcast as being an essential part of the Christian mission to the souls of men and women. It was largely for this reason that its power has become a permanent feature in modern English life. It does not depend upon revivalism alone."[65]

William Booth's theology of personhood prioritized the eternal life of the soul above the body but he appreciated the importance of the body—unlike some evangelists of the time who prioritized the soul to the exclusion of the body. However, Booth experienced tensions sustaining a unity of body-soul and often resorted to a "soul priority" argument when defending the development of social work against those who suggested it marked a dilution or deviation from the Army's evangelical message. For example, in the foreword to *In Darkest England*, Booth is unequivocal: "I must assert in the most unqualified way that it is primarily and mainly for the sake of saving the soul that I seek the salvation of the body."[66] In similar vein, William Booth prioritized the saving of souls in the social service programs. In a letter to all officers a few years before his death, he devotes a paragraph to the officers working in the social agencies and instructs them:

---

65. Sandall, *The History of the Salvation Army, Volume Three,* xiii.
66. Booth, *In Darkest England,* xiv.

> Do all the good you can to the bodies and circumstances of the unhappy and restless wanderers who come under your influence ... But while you strive to deliver them from their temporal distresses and endeavor to rescue them from the causes that have led to their unfortunate condition, you must seek, above all, to turn their miseries to good account by making them help the salvation of their souls and their deliverance from the wrath to come. It will be a very small reward for all your toils if, after bringing them into conditions of well-being here, they perish hereafter.[67]

William Booth appears to have moved away from John Wesley's holistic conception of health and personhood. In his sermon "The Image of God," Wesley emphasized the wholeness of the original created order: "With Adam it was ordained by the original law that during this vital union neither part of the compound should act at all but together with its companion; that the dependence of each upon the other should be inviolably maintained ... While Adam's sin did introduce disorder and dis-ease into the original creation, it did not interrupt the vital union between body and soul."[68]

As E. Brooks Holifield observes, "Precisely because he could not accept a dualistic severing of the soul from the body in the original creation, Wesley had to assume that body and soul remained interdependent after the Fall. Consequently, the body is not to be viewed as a 'a second class citizen.'"[69] Despite William Booth's concern for the physical condition of the poorest people and his Wesleyan heritage of an integrated body-soul, he appears to view the body as "second class." Catherine Booth—the theologian in the Booths' partnership—appears, at times, to endorse an orthodox Wesleyan concept of salvation effecting a healing and restoration with implications for the entire created order. In a sermon in 1881, Catherine asserted: "It is not a scheme of salvation merely—it is a scheme of restoration. He proposes to restore me—brain, heart, soul, spirit, body, every fibre of my nature to restore me perfectly, to conform me wholly to the image of his Son."[70]

However, at other times, Catherine also tended to struggle to keep body and soul together—and she tended to prioritize the soul. In a

---

67. Idem., *A Letter from the General*, 44.
68. Wesley, *The Works of John Wesley*, 296.
69. Source: Ott, "John Wesley on Health as Wholeness," 44.
70. Booth, *Godliness*, 165.

sermon preached in the summer of 1880, Catherine Booth took as her text Ephesians 5:18, "Be filled with the Spirit." She argued: "The very essence and core of religion is God first and allegiance and obedience to him first... if I cannot keep my health and be faithful to Him, then I must sacrifice it... if I cannot keep my life and be faithful to Him, then I must be prepared to lose it and lay my neck on the block if need be... That is my religion and I do not know any other."[71]

Barbara Robinson argues the early Salvationists view of the soul and the temporal nature of the body led to an undervaluing of personal health. The Salvationist culture, driven by triumphalist, postmillennial expectations, started to expect that saved souls would sacrifice their physical wellbeing in the cause of saving other souls. "A perfected body was not the physiological equivalent of a perfected soul... health was a proximate rather than absolute good, desirable as a source of adequate strength and necessary energy for the fulfillment of duty."[72]

A focus on personal sanctification, I contend, was based on an individualistic conception of holiness that emphasized a differentiation between the pure and the impure. This enabled the development of dual mission for corps (soul work) and social services (body work). The establishment of dual organizational structures for corps and social services embedded a duality into Salvation Army practice resulting in the delinking of congregations (corps) from a rapidly professionalizing social work operation. Although justified on the grounds of pragmatic organizational management, the dividing of The Salvation Army between corps and social was influenced, at least in part, by a theological dualism of personhood.

In the century since the death of William Booth, Salvationist theological anthropology has been in a state of flux. On two occasions The Salvation Army's Eleven Articles of Faith[73] refer to "body" and "soul" and the Ninth Article quotes directly from 1 Thessalonians 5:23 with the phrase "body, soul, and spirit." I have noted a number of my contemporaries describing persons as "body, soul, and spirit" despite there being

---

71. Idem., "Filled with the Spirit," 3–4.
72. Robinson, "Bodily Compassion," 18.
73. The Salvation Army, *Salvation Story*, 85 and 115.

little Scriptural support for a tri-partite anthropology of the person nor has any such formulation gained credence in the history of the Church.[74]

Salvation Army official teaching on the nature of human persons has developed over the past century. For example, the 1923 edition of the *Handbook of Doctrine* adopts the rationality argument in its teaching on personhood: "Man, as we see and know him, is ONE BEING, YET HE HAS BOTH A BODY AND A SOUL, or a lower and higher nature" (*emphasis in original*).[75] By the 1998 version, there is hardly a mention of body and soul[76] and much greater emphasis on the Trinity as relational and some references to the relationality of persons.[77] The recently published 2010 version of the *Handbook of Doctrine* retains the relationality teaching and adds an explicit rejection of body-soul dualism: "In Salvationist faith and practice the wholeness of the person is crucial. It is reflected in the combination of our evangelistic and social work. The (eleventh) doctrine (eschatology) underlines this wholeness as we believe in a resurrection of our total being . . . Any dualistic thinking which separates body and soul, often suggesting the body is either less important or evil, must be resisted as it can lead to unhealthy or immoral practice. Salvationist teaching must clearly present the wholeness of the individual as a basis for personal spiritual life and mission in the world."[78]

In summary, a priority for the soul over the body impacted Salvation Army practice. It was exacerbated by an emphasis on individual sanctification that led to greater separation between corps and social institution, contributing to the fragmentation of Salvation Army mission.

Booth's Mission

Some have argued the publication of *In Darkest England* marks a change of direction in Booth's thinking and the birth of a "dual mission" for The

---

74. Maddox notes that John Wesley struggled with the Scriptural reference to a tri-partite anthropology but "for all intents and purposes Wesley assumed a two-dimensional anthropology." Maddox, *Responsible Grace*, 71.

75. The Salvation Army, *Handbook of Salvation Army Doctrine*, 44.

76. The 1998 version collapses all differentiation between body and soul with the assertion: "In the Bible the word "body" means the whole person. The phrase safeguards the integrity of the human person" (118).

77. The Salvation Army, *Salvation Story*, 60.

78. Idem., *The Salvation Army Handbook of Doctrine*, 243.

Salvation Army.[79] Walker argues the shaping of a "dual mission of evangelizing and social services" began in 1884.[80] The "dual mission" frame has gained credence both within historical assessments of Booth's Salvation Army[81] and in contemporary understandings of Salvation Army mission. Although William Booth used the term "dual mission," as argued in the previous section, his *telos* was always theological and any dualism among early Salvation Army practice arose not simply because of a separation of evangelism and humanitarianism but due to a dualistic construction of personhood. Booth's commitment to social engagement began soon after his conversion when he became involved working with homeless people. It was not an "1890 addendum."[82] Secular historians such as Roy Hattersley agree that Booth justified his mission on theological rather than ideological grounds.[83]

Admittedly, the evidence is not clear-cut. In a history of Salvation Army social work, John Coutts notes that "on this relationship between men's spiritual and social needs William Booth was not wholly consistent."[84] Ann Woodall argues that at times Booth described personal and social salvation as two sides of the same coin but, at other times, he spoke of social redemption as a way to make it easier for people to accept personal redemption.[85] Despite inconsistency in his use of terms like "second mission"—probably the result of his pragmatic activism—Booth repeatedly refused to accept a dualist soteriology and rejected any salvation of the body without the salvation of the soul. As Woodall notes, Booth's mission was always integrated—"social work was religious and religious work was social."[86] Booth may have developed a more complete appreciation of God's soteriological purposes during his lifetime but this

---

79. Keating, *Into Unknown England*, 19. Murdoch, *Origins of the Salvation Army*, 113.

80. Walker, *Pulling the Devil's Kingdom Down*, 239.

81. Himmelfarb, *Poverty and Compassion*, 222. Dibble, "The Salvation Army—the Search of a Wholistic Ministry," 1. Dibble who begins with the statement: "For 100 years, The Salvation Army has had a dual mission: to bring men and women into right relationship with God through its evangelism and to improve their physical condition through its social work."

82. Woodall, *What Price the Poor?*, 162.

83. Hattersley, *Blood and Fire*, 355.

84. Coutts, *The Salvationists*, 19.

85. Woodall, *What Price the Poor?*, 166.

86. Ibid., 164.

should not be read as a sustained dualism of evangelism and humanitarianism. More importantly, it does not justify a dual *telos* in the contemporary Salvation Army.

For example, on his 81st birthday in 1910, Booth responded to a journalist who suggested he had said rehabilitation of religion would come along the line of social service: "That is only partly true. Social service is only the expression of life, which abides in the soul and forces into activity the desire to take upon oneself the burdens of humanity. It is only when we get more soul into our lives that we are able to do any good . . . All the social activity of the Army is the outcome of the spiritual life of its members. All social service must be based on the spiritual, or it will amount to little in the end."[87]

I will return to this issue later as it highlights a critically important question for Salvation Army health ministry: Can a common *telos* be sought by all parts of The Salvation Army or is a "dual mission" a more faithful conception of Salvation Army ministry?

Booth's Eschatological Telos

Roger Green argues Booth's missiology and eschatological *telos* was influenced by post-millennialism[88] because, in his latter years, Booth wanted Salvationists to understand the "dual mission" in the light of his unified theology of redemption: "The dual mission of the Army, undergirded by a theology of redemption that was both personal and social, was preparatory to the establishment of the millennial kingdom on earth and thereby a harbinger of the Second Advent of Christ . . . And, in Booth's mind, he and his Army were the center of that salvation story."[89]

Booth's clearest articulation of his eschatology is contained in articles published in *All The World*, an internal publication, in 1889[90] and 1890[91]—around the time *In Darkest England* was being written. Booth's eschatology depended on two key beliefs. Firstly, the establishment of

---

87. Sandall, *The History of the Salvation Army, Volume Three*, xiv.

88. Post-millennialists believe the millennium comes first (usually as evidence of present Christian agencies at work in the world) and the Second Coming will occur at the end of process. I thank Major Wendy Swan, a Canadian Salvation Army officer and a doctoral student at King's College London for her guidance on this section.

89. Green, *The Life and Ministry of William Booth*, 206.

90. Booth, "Salvation for Both Worlds," 1–6.

91. Idem., "The Millenium," 337–43.

the Kingdom of God on Earth was part of the work of redemption and the triumph over evil. Secondly, The Salvation Army had been chosen by God as the chief instrument in bringing about God's Kingdom on Earth. Booth believed that just as God willed an individual could enjoy full salvation so God extended that will to the whole world. He did not set a time frame for the Millennium but wanted Salvationists to understand their part. However, Booth believed God's kingdom was primarily a spiritual kingdom and could not be ushered in or sustained by human effort apart from God. In *In Darkest England*, Booth wrote: "I am labouring under no delusions as to the possibility of inaugurating the Millennium by any social specific."[92]

This enthusiastic eschatology resulted in The Salvation Army giving little attention to ecclesiology. If God had chosen The Salvation Army as his chief instrument for the bringing about of the Kingdom, the relationship with the Church was, therefore, not a priority. Consequentially, Salvation Army ecclesiology remained officially undefined for almost another century.[93] Booth's Salvationists shed "churchy" baggage when they believed it hindered the mission. By 1890, The Salvation Army had stopped observing the sacraments of Eucharist and Baptism. This was not a move towards a secular eschatology—as Plant identified in contemporary FBO practice.[94] Rather the early Salvationists embraced an eschatological imperialism for the purpose of "saving the world" empowered by the Holy Spirit through dutifully participating in practices of worship such as preaching, prayer, singing, brass bands, and nightly meetings. Booth presumed Salvation Army social work institutions and colonies would include Salvation Army corps (congregations). Booth did not make worship a condition of participation in any social program but argued Salvation Army worship should be so attractive people would not want to miss it. He placed the onus on Salvationists to attract people into the Kingdom rather than use coercive methods.[95]

---

92. Idem., *In Darkest England*, 44.

93. The Salvation Army's ecclesiology has received significant attention in the past two decades from senior Salvation Army leaders culminating in the inclusion of an ecclesiological statement in the 2010 edition of *The Salvation Army Handbook of Doctrine* entitled "The Salvation Army in the Body of Christ." *The Salvation Army Handbook of Doctrine*, 310–18.

94. Plant, "International Development and Belief in Progress," 849.

95. Booth, *In Darkest England*, 139.

The conclusion to be drawn is that Booth and the early Salvationists were orientated by an eschatological *telos*, shaped by a post-millennial eschatology with overtones of Victorian England imperialism. However, in seeking an eschatological *telos* for Salvation Army health ministry I seek to build on Salvation Army tradition—albeit seeking to move towards a more appropriate eschatological *telos* for today's post-colonial world. In Chapter 5, I will seek to articulate a more faithful eschatological *telos* for twenty-first century Salvation Army health ministry.

The Salvation Army in the World

Booth's manifesto for social change, coupled with the rapid growth of The Salvation Army in the UK and beyond, unsettled and intrigued the British establishment. Booth attracted the ire of Professor Huxley—a colleague of Charles Darwin—who, soon after the publication of *In Darkest England*, engaged in a campaign through the letters page of *The Times* newspaper to discredit Booth's plan. Huxley had three main criticisms of the Booths—the autocratic style of governance in The Salvation Army; the outcome was likely to denigrate and subjugate people rather than progress the individual; the funds and property of The Salvation Army was benefiting the Booths at the expense of hard-working officers.[96] Underpinning Huxley's critique was his dislike of Booth's individualistic, evangelical soteriology. Lawson developed a helpful analysis of *The Times* discussion that stretched over several weeks at the end of 1890.[97] He summarizes: "Huxley called Booth's system "autocratic socialism" masked by its theological exterior. He provided case histories, which, he claimed, showed the Booth's autocratic form of government lacked basic Christian compassion. Huxley also raised serious questions regarding Booth's integrity in respect of the money and property of The Salvation Army which was held "in trust" by William Booth."[98]

Booth agreed to a committee of inquiry led by Earl Onslow (former Governor of New Zealand) assisted by five other eminent members. Eighteen meetings were held and the 69-page report published on 2

---

96. Lawson, "William Booth's Darkest England Scheme," 27–28.

97. It is interesting to note the extent to which Lawson, a Salvation Army officer, accepts the premise that Booth's soul-saving motivation should not color the work of saving the bodies. It suggests the extent to which dualist orientations have embedded in Salvation Army practice.

98. Lawson, "William Booth's Darkest England Scheme," 22.

December 1892 exonerated Booth and The Salvation Army of any misappropriation.[99] However, this welter of public attention impacted The Salvation Army significantly resulting in Booth creating a separate trust for social work—distinct from evangelical work—a dichotomy that continues to encourage the fragmentation of Salvation Army engagement in the world.

Booth's acceptance of the financial fragmentation of The Salvation Army was indicative of an increasing reticence to engage in controversy. Salvationists perceived the established denominations were deflected from God's work of redeeming the world by needless disputes. George Scott Railton, the most influential Salvation Army leader outside of the Booth family, argued a non-confrontation approach was key to the Army's inter-cultural expansion: "The one-mindedness and one-heartedness of The Army is strikingly exemplified in its newspapers and its prayers. It has 61 publications, issued in 49 different countries and colonies, in 23 different languages. In not one of these can there be found any recognition of the controversies, which disturb the Christian world. They represent minds always engaged upon one subject—the subjugation of the world to the dominion of Jesus Christ."[100]

This non-confrontational approach also characterized relations with the state and wider society. Diane Winston argues that once the perceived threat of The Salvation Army to the established religious and secular order had passed, people became largely indifferent to any teleological influences in Salvation Army practice. Winston argues the decision to avoid controversy—theological and political—enabled The Salvation Army to offer up a kind of blank slate or "canvas" for religious projection.[101]

I am not convinced this was ever the intention of the early Salvationist leaders. Such a "blank canvas approach" would make The Salvation Army particularly vulnerable to the forces of isomorphism and the founders were acutely aware of the challenge of keeping the Army soteriologically orientated. For example, William Booth's instruction to his officers on party politics in 1891 presents a constructive appreciation of the function of the state while emphasizing the distinctive agenda of the people of God.

99. Ibid., 29.
100. Railton, *The Salvation Army Following Christ*, 195.
101. Winston, *Red-Hot and Righteous*.

> The relation of The Army to Governments is determined by the principle that we are not of this world and therefore cannot be expected to feel any deep interest in those governments which exclusively belong to it and which are conducted without any regard to the will of God and the interests of his Kingdom . . . If any political party is supported with a view to the making or carrying out of some good law, our special co-operation with that party must cease with the accomplishment of the end desired. Our policy is measures, not parties and only such measures as are directly favorable to the Salvation and well being of the people.[102]

In relations with the state, William Booth had a remarkably expansive and confident vision for the impact of The Salvation Army across the world. He was willing to engage with the two dominant political visions of the age—imperialism and socialism—but responded with an eschatological *telos* with priority to God's kingdom rather than taking ideological sides. Bebbington argues the willingness of evangelicals to partner with the colonialists was linked to their understanding of sin: "There was, after the last years of the nineteenth century, less compunction about expansion and more expectation of the benefits from colonial rule. Hence evangelicals became more enthusiastic about the moral possibilities of British power abroad . . . Empire, like atonement, came to be seen as a means of redeeming human beings from slavery to sin."[103]

Although it was not the intention of the early Salvationist leaders to offer their Salvation Army up as a blank slate for external projection, the characteristic of non-confrontation began to characterize relations with the forces of market and state making it a far cry from Evers' proposal for a "civilized culture of conflict."[104] The following section describes the development of Salvation Army social services in the years after the publication of *In Darkest England* revealing a number of tensions that emerged as the scheme was implemented.

THE IMPACT OF IN DARKEST ENGLAND—REFLECTING ON 1911 AND 1921 SOCIAL COUNCILS

The publication of *In Darkest England* initiated a global experiment in social policy by The Salvation Army with the expansion of an institutionally

---

102. The Salvation Army, *Orders and Regulations for Field Officers*, 243.
103. Bebbington, "Atonement, Sun and Empire 1880 to 1914," 243–44.
104. Evers, "Part of the Welfare Mix," 167.

based mission footprint. Spontaneous responses to social problems by Salvationists in their neighborhoods were replaced with institutionally based social work increasingly undertaken by paid professionals. William Booth was aware of the dangers of losing the soul-saving character of The Salvation Army. Begbie argues that as early as 1898 Booth "began, if not to lose faith in the efficacy of social reform, at least to question whether he had done wisely in throwing so much of his energy into this tremendous struggle."[105] Pamela Walker argues: "[The Salvation Army] was no longer pulling the devil's kingdom down with brass bands playing music hall tunes, fiery preachers, and processions through working-class neighborhoods. Instead it became a religious sect with a social service wing that was often the more vibrant and prominent half, creating strong ties to other Christian and state-run agencies."[106]

In an attempt to identify changes in practice, I reviewed the records of two international gatherings of Salvationist social ministry practitioners held in London 20 years and 30 years respectively after the publication of *In Darkest England.* In a keynote address at the 1911 International Social Council—just a year before his death, William Booth presents a much clearer articulation of the faithful characteristics of Salvation Army social ministry than he presented *In Darkest England*: "Those operations of The Salvation Army which have to do with the alleviation, or removal, of the moral and temporal evils which cause so much of the misery of the submerged classes and which so greatly hinders their Salvation. Our Social Operations, thus defined, are the natural outcome of Salvationism, or I might say of Christianity, as instituted, described, proclaimed, and exemplified in the life, teaching, and sacrifices of Jesus Christ."[107]

Booth was not reticent in claiming significant status for Salvation Army social work. Although he acknowledges there has always been social work but he claims "Social Work, as a . . . department of the Kingdom of Jesus Christ, recognized, organized, and provided for, had to wait for The Salvation Army . . . It can neither be contemplated, commenced, nor carried on, with any great success, without a heart full of pity, and love, and endued with the power of the Holy Ghost."[108]

---

105. Begbie, *Life of William Booth*, 142.
106. Walker, *Pulling the Devil's Kingdom Down*, 264.
107. Booth, *The Principles of Social Work*, 1.
108. Ibid., 18.

Booth is alert to the dangers of employing people who do not share the same convictions arguing there would have been "considerably more doleful failures than those we have experienced."[109] Booth set out the characteristics of a social officer—"compassion; aggression; wisdom; justice; self-sacrifice; warm-heartedness" but without these, "he will be comparatively useless and, more or less, a sorrowful failure."[110] These are, for Booth, the characteristics of the Salvation soldier, the result of a clear eschatological orientation developed through the process of salvation and sanctification rather than a common set of skills available to everyone.

Booth emphasized the importance of synergy between the Salvation Army's two departments—social (institutions) and field (congregations)—but he is careful to stress the unity and resists any hint of dualism in soteriology.

> Although distinct in their character and different in their modes of operation, these two great departments, the Social and Field, constitute one and the same Organization. These departments may be regarded as the two sides of one great whole; or, to use another figure, they may be compared to a right and left hand, each hand distinct from the other, one doing work more readily and effectively in one direction, while the other performs work of a superior value in another direction and yet both of incomparable value, each being unable to say to the other, "I have no need of thee" but take the two in combination and you have the one Salvation Army.[111]

Senior leaders speaking at the 1911 also voiced concern at the risks of Salvation Army social work losing its faith-based character. Commissioner Howard resisted the notion that "work is worship" and urged social officers not to use this as an "excuse for the neglect of spiritual exercises and for the absence of those special relations to God that are so essential."[112] It is notable that the leaders of the now non-Eucharistic Salvation Army were particularly insistent regarding the importance of spiritual exercises in sustaining the faithfulness of the person and the ministry. Howard also criticized the notion of "The Professional Officer"

---

109. Ibid., 19.
110. Ibid., 41.
111. Ibid., 62.
112. Howard, "Spiritual Standards," 218.

and urged his listeners "that the fire must be kept burning and the passion must be cultivated."[113]

Edward Higgins—who later became the third Salvation Army General in 1929—gave a lengthy lecture in 1911 on unity. He noted the strengths in the diversity of Salvation Army social operations but also notes the risks of division. "While we insist upon the Fatherhood of God for every branch, we also insist that it must be the same Army, with its one government, and with the same unchanging and undiluted principles."[114] Higgins argued for a teleological unity amid the diversity of operations:

> Without a fixed object for which we are all working, the results of our labors will be anything but harmonious. Certainly the purpose should be the advancement of the glory of God and the furtherance of his interests on earth; and as Salvationists we believe that this can be most quickly effected by the establishment of The Army and the raising up of a force of men and women who will fight beneath its Colors and pledge themselves to its principles. The design of the Social Officer should be the making of Salvation Soldiers—that purpose should be placed first amongst the many others he may have and all the others should be made to bend to this one.[115]

However, despite Booth and Higgins' articulation of a shared *telos*, the 1921 international social work conference opened in London with a Social Work Pageant in the Royal Albert Hall suggesting a different priority. The official report suggests an alternative *telos* was beginning to take hold—an orientation towards the development of people as "good citizens of society."[116] The reporter noted the pageant showed "derelict men taken from prison, street, and the dens of the destitute, placed in elevators, given good work, and hope, and finally, as citizens of value to their community, passed out to achieve in the ordinary walks of life."[117] The men were given "good work and hope" without any explicit reference to Christocentric soteriology.

In contrast to the message of the pageant, Bramwell Booth, who became General after the death of William in 1912, echoed his father's

113. Ibid., 220.
114. Higgins, "Unity of Operations," 1.
115. Ibid., 6.
116. The Salvation Army, "The International Social Council," xi.
117. Ibid.

arguments a decade earlier in emphasizing the unity of the Army and the common objective "to spread the Salvation of God, and the making of men and women into the disciples of His Son Jesus Christ."[118] He repeatedly voiced concern about fragmentation noting "persons responsible for the different sections tend too much to separate themselves from other sections."[119] One example of this was people being saved through the ministry of the social operations not being accepted into the corps.[120] However, Bramwell offered no structural changes or common processes to overcome the process of fragmentation. If anything, he appeared to make the situation worse. He demanded social services raise up its own officers and not rely on officers sent to the officer training college from the corps. He used language unlikely to heal the fractures stating: "I deplore the extent to which the Social Work has become a parasite in this matter all over the world."[121] In another reference Bramwell suggests the social work is not part of the "proper" Army: "The ultimate success of the Social Work must more and more be measured by the extent to which men and women and children are brought to the knowledge of Salvation and passed on to The Army."[122]

Tensions regarding the popularity of the social work and its ability to attract funding were already emerging. Bramwell acknowledged that social work is "attractive to the world and that even the basest worldlings are compelled to admit that this work is worthy of support."[123] Bramwell warned against accepting money that cannot be properly used "lest it should become a curse rather than a blessing"[124] and highlighted sources of pressures that needed to be resisted. He said, "No influence of any kind—religious, national, municipal, commercial, or political—must affect the character of the humanitarian effort which we are making for the benefit of the people." Bramwell did not go on to identify processes and practices to resist these pressures.[125]

118. Booth, "The General's Address," 34.
119. Ibid.
120. A corps is a Salvation Army worshipping congregation.
121. Booth, "The General's Address," 34.
122. Ibid., 36.
123. Ibid.
124. Ibid., 46.
125. Ibid., 47.

THE LEGACY OF IN DARKEST ENGLAND

Woodall argues a key factor in the success of William Booth was his combination of a theology of the atonement and sanctification with the social conscience of incarnational theology. Woodall notes that Booth saw Jesus as an example, in the light of incarnational theology, but he never saw him as only an example: "He would never preach about Jesus without preaching of him as Saviour. If his entry into social work was interpreted as an increased emphasis on the Incarnation, it was never for Booth at the cost of less emphasis on the Atonement... If there was any major difference in his theology it was not a shift or change of direction but a broadening to include the idea of social redemption and then not so much an ideological change, more an acceptance of the Army's work within that plan."[126]

Woodall argues this tension between atonement, sanctification, and incarnational theology resulted in The Salvation Army retaining a flexibility and adaptability. Booth's insistence on the centrality of the atonement prevented The Salvation Army's drift into "merely being an ineffectual social agency."[127] By failing to resolve the tensions between the atonement-sanctification doctrine of the evangelical Salvation Army and the social engagement of Incarnational theology, "[Booth] quite unknowingly, helped to prevent his organization becoming locked in a time warp and being only applicable in certain areas and cultures. The tensions were creative ones that gave it the impetus to adapt. Its commitment to social reclamation prevented it from becoming marginalized as a corybantic sect while its evangelical theology prevented it from being lost in a diffusive, social Christianity that was ripe to be taken over by the welfare state."[128]

I wish to take Woodall's argument further. Not only did a tension in Booth's doctrines of atonement, sanctification, and incarnation keep The Salvation Army faithful; critically, the habits and practices of worship, filled with the Spirit and orientated by an eschatological *telos* sustained the faithful presence of Salvationists in the world. The experience of being faithfully present in the world enriched Salvation Army worship. Lives changed, habits altered, and relationships were strengthened. In particular, the sharing of personal testimony became a characteristic

---

126. Woodall, *What Price the Poor?*, 167.
127. Ibid.
128. Ibid., 168–69.

of Salvation Army worship and an example of its practical theology. Theology shaped practice and practice shaped theology—all orientated by an eschatological *telos*.

However, a united *telos* was not sustained throughout The Salvation Army. The *Darkest England* scheme resulted in increased publicity for Booth's work resulting in social work becoming more institutionalized and "professionalized."[129] Woodall argues that as the years passed The Salvation Army's involvement in social work "led it to abandon its evangelical theological stance in favour of a more liberal incarnationalism" with the result it was no longer a threat to the religious or secular authorities but began to work within the existing system.[130] Woodall's analysis is important. As Salvation Army social work became more established the incarnational theology of "being with" the poor replaced the postmillennial theology of "going for souls and going for the worst." As a result, The Salvation Army moved through the twentieth century with a fragmented theology: corps prioritized on atonement and sanctification; social services programs embraced a liberal incarnationalism which lacked theological resilience as the social services came under an increasing pressure from secularist funders to "professionalize." Over time, the gap left by the demise of atonement theology in social services was filled by a humanitarian eschatology.

I am, to some extent, over-stating the demise of theology in Salvation Army practice. Diane Winston and Charles Glenn's research suggests the Salvation Army's theology has, over the years, assisted in resisting the isomorphic forces to some degree.[131] However, whatever the degree of unfaithfulness in Salvation Army practice, implicit in Glenn, Woodall, and Winston's reflections is an acknowledgment of the contribution theology makes in achieving faithful practice.

PHILIP NEEDHAM'S ATTEMPT TO ADDRESS THE TENSIONS

This practical theological reflection on Salvation Army health ministry seeks insights from Salvation Army experience to inform future practice. This chapter has focused on the early years of The Salvation Army (1865 to 1921) but now reflects on more recent practice. I engage with Philip

---

129. Ibid., 162.
130. Ibid., 211.
131. Winston, *Red-Hot and Righteous*, 49.

Needham—one of the most influential voices in Salvation Army theology and missiology in the past 25 years. Needham was an influential member of the International Doctrine Council that revised the Salvation Army Doctrine Book in the late 1990s[132] and was a key adviser to the working group that developed the *Mission in Community* workbook in 2005.[133] In addition, Needham has written a number of articles that provide insights into contemporary Salvation Army theology and practice.[134] Needham has responded to a number of the tensions identified in the previous section. I will highlight a number of these points and identify areas for further reflection.

The Salvation Army, the Church, and a Common Telos

The ecclesiological ambiguity created by William Booth continued through Salvation Army life in the twentieth century. Needham wrote *Community in Mission* in 1987 to answer the following question: "From a Salvationist perspective, how are we to understand who the people of God are and what their purpose in the world is?"[135] Needham acknowledges a scarcity of theological tools in The Salvation Army: "The Army is seriously in need of developing theological tools with which to be discriminating and responsible in its warfare. This is not a plea for spending more time on the finer points of theology. It is a plea for the development of an ongoing theology of mission informed both by Scriptures and tradition and by the contemporary situation."[136]

Needham articulates a distinctive ecclesial character for The Salvation Army moving away from any special "post-millennial" status and situating The Salvation Army firmly within the wider Christian Church. Needham stated:

> The Salvation Army—as this movement came to be called in 1878—is as much an integral part of the one true catholic (universal) Christian Church as any other denomination or ecclesiastical tradition . . . It has no right to claim ecclesiastical superiority.

---

132. The Salvation Army, *Salvation Story*.

133. Idem., *Mission in Community*.

134. Needham, "Towards a Re-Integration of the Salvationist Mission," Needham, "The Theology," Needham, "Integrating Holiness and Community."

135. Needham, *Community in Mission*, 5.

136. Ibid., 74.

> Like any other denomination, it has its strengths and weaknesses. It has not always maintained its missionary commitment and it has at times been guilty of spiritual Phariseeism. It has sometimes displayed an isolationist and sectarian spirit. And it has suffered some of the deadly consequences of creeping institutionalization. The Salvation Army is no better—or worse—than its sister fellowships in Christ.[137]

Needham's response is to articulate a Salvationist ecclesiology around six key points. He begins each point with "The Church" in a clear move to position The Salvation Army within the body of Christ. Firstly, "The Church is a community which comes into being in response to the Kingdom of God through faith in Jesus Christ as the one in whom the Kingdom is realized."[138] Secondly, "The Church is a fellowship created by the Holy Spirit in which those who have responded to the Kingdom of God through faith are empowered to live redemptive lives."[139] Thirdly, "The Church is a band of pilgrims who are called to separate themselves from the oppressive patterns of the present world order and to keep moving towards the possibilities which the new Kingdom in Christ offers."[140] Fourthly, "The Church is an army which exists for the purpose of fighting every enslavement to sin, disarming the causes of human oppression, and overcoming obstacles to pilgrimage."[141] Fifthly, "The Church is a gathered community in which the missionary people of God encourage one another's spiritual growth and equip one another for mission."[142] Sixthly, "The Church is the eschatological community that prays for the coming Kingdom and lives in the light of its dawning."[143]

Needham is not primarily concerned about positioning Salvationists within the Church. His prime concern is the breakdown of relations between the Christian Church (including The Salvation Army) and society. Although Needham uses dualistic terms to describe Salvation Army mission—social action and evangelism—he explains social action as "not merely charitable acts towards those who are outside the fellowship.

137. Ibid., 2–3.
138. Ibid., 6.
139. Ibid., 14.
140. Ibid., 35.
141. Ibid., 52.
142. Ibid., 75.
143. Ibid., 91.

Rather, they are the "overflow" of Christian caring within that fellowship . . . In carrying out its mission, the Church is actually embodying not so much what it thinks it should do, but what it is."[144] Needham identifies the importance of an eschatological *telos* for the Christian church—and particularly The Salvation Army: "[The church] must demonstrate the future so it can point the world to its future. It is the eschatological community that not only *prays* for the Kingdom to come but also *lives* in the light of its dawning . . . The Church prays and lives as a colony of hope that is committed to the coming future in Christ."[145]

Tensions over The Salvation Army's place in the church reduced further culminating in an official statement in 2008 clarifying the place of The Salvation Army in the body of Christ.[146]

Articulating a Theology of Health, Healing, and Wholeness

Needham also made a substantial contribution to the articulation of a Salvation Army theology of health ministry. He argues for a central place for health, healing, and wholeness in the life and mission of the Church.

> Health, healing, and wholeness are central concerns in the life and mission of the Church . . . They are indispensable to understanding the Church's mission. Every Christian is called to experience personal healing, to participate in corporate healing and to represent Christ's healing power in the world . . . It is basic to everything the Church is and does. The Church is made up of those who know the healing force of sins forgiven (Psalm 30:2; 103:3; Luke 4:18; John 12:40; Acts 10:30; 1 Peter 2:24); who are experiencing the healing of relationships (Ephesians 2:11–22); and who are called to be agents of healing (2 Corinthians 5:15–21; James 5:13–16; Acts 5:16).[147]

Needham develops three arguments. Firstly, the Church proclaims a gospel that heals. Secondly, the Church's mission is to bring healing to individuals as well as to nations. Thirdly, the church's own congregations are called to be centers of healing.[148] In developing these arguments he

---

144. Needham, *Community in Mission*, 64–65.
145. Ibid., 92.
146. The Salvation Army, *Salvationist Ecclesiological Statement*.
147. Needham, "The Theology," 25.
148. Ibid. 25–65.

addresses a number of theological weaknesses I have noted in Salvation Army practice. Firstly, Needham emphasizes a relational appreciation of personhood and highlights the nature of the creator Trinitarian God who is "a person in relationship"[149] and created people in his image. Needham dismisses the priority of "soul" over "body" as a dangerous dualism because "the soul is seen as good and the body as evil or temporary" which can result in "physical suffering being disparaged," "bodily health can be ignored" or the "body can be indulged or abused."[150] Secondly, Needham rejects a "theology of eschatological postponement . . . that gives rise to shallow, short-term, non-relational, care" and calls for Salvation Army healing ministry to "take place in the context of a hopeful future" and be "inclusive of the whosoever and appreciate the interconnectedness of life."[151] Needham rejects a short-term fixing of the body and promotes an appreciation of the integrated nature of people.

Prioritizing Pneumatology and Problematizing Institutions

Both Booth and Needham identify a fallen, fragmented world in need of redemption. Booth offers his scheme complete with a mechanistic, institutional solution for poverty all around the world. In the 100 years since *In Darkest England*, The Salvation Army prioritized the development of institutions with the acquisition of many properties. Needham, living with the outcome of institutional atrophy, expresses fears of being "tied down to the static structures and the stubborn status quos of this world."[152] Needham appears as resistant to institutional solutions as Booth is committed to them. Needham calls on Salvationists to embark on mission into community and he uses the image of a "caravan." However, Needham does not explain how to transform Booth's "colonies" and "citadels" into "caravans." Needham appears to ignore the legacy of Booth's grand scheme in his proposals.

Needham goes further in negatively linking tradition and ritual with institutional self-preservation. With overtones of sacramental skepticism, Needham contrasts "the word of God" with the traditions of the church. "A Church on the move has more need for leaders who will discern and

---

149. Ibid. 29.
150. Ibid. 37.
151. Ibid., 33–34.
152. Idem., *Community in Mission*, 37.

speak the word of God than for those who will maintain the traditions."¹⁵³ Needham views religious habits and traditions through the lens of ecclesiastical hierarchy and disempowered laity. Needham's unease with the traditionalism and institutionalization of The Salvation Army leads him to priorities "process" over "form" and he argues: "A Salvationist ecclesiology holds that everything connected with the ordering of the Church's life and work must serve its missionary calling. One important way to build structures that serve the Church's mission is to emphasize process rather than form. It is far more crucial to preserve the process that has shaped a missionary tradition than the forms which that process has created . . . The spiritual truth that death must come before life applies to institutions as well as persons."¹⁵⁴

With the benefit of hindsight, I am not convinced by Needham's promotion of a de-institutionalized mission with priority for process over form. I contend there does not need to be a choice between process and form. More important is the extent to which process and/or form contribute to the task of restoring fractured relationships. Both process and form can be orientated towards building deeper relationships with a *telos* of "healthy persons." Needham introduces a dualism into Salvationist ecclesiology—between process and form—which has been unhelpful. This distinction has been used by some well-meaning, but misguided, Salvationists in recent years to deconstruct the habits and institutions of The Salvation Army without appreciating the importance of replacing them with repositories of resilient, embedded, faithful habits, and practices. Therefore, I am hesitant to endorse a de-institutional approach to Salvation Army health ministry, particularly in light of the current anti-institutional trend that is signaling an exodus from congregational life.¹⁵⁵ Institutions, traditions, and habits are not intrinsically oppositional to the work of the Spirit. As will be argued in the next chapter, they can be rightly orientated by an eschatological *telos*.

The Value of Community

Needham's vision for The Salvation Army moving from "colonies" to "caravans" was complicated by a blurring of his definition of "community."

---

153. Ibid., 42.
154. Ibid., 57.
155. Hunter, *To Change the World*, 283.

To evidence this assertion, I refer to a paper delivered by Needham in 2000 in which he presents an insightful critique of the contemporary practice of holiness in The Salvation Army. Helpfully, he begins arguing that "at this time in our history, it is crucial for Salvationists to understand and live the corporate dimensions of holiness and to develop an ecclesiology grounded in the call to holiness."[156] Needham voiced four concerns. Firstly, Salvationist commitment to "the radical concepts of a holy lifestyle"[157] seems weaker than earlier days. Secondly, the ecclesiology debate in The Salvation Army should resist being driven by sociology rather than by theology.[158] Thirdly, The Salvation Army is "under the spell of Western individualism" to the extent that "we focus on our individual relationship with God and what God can do in our lives personally. We say far less about how God works in community and our own relationships in community."[159] Fourthly, Salvationists see the relationship between holiness and community as one-directional. "I do not think that the relationship between holiness and community is simply one-directional. Holiness is also nurtured by community and is meaningless apart from it . . . We need to do more work in articulating the important role of community in shaping our holiness."[160]

Needham makes many excellent and helpful points in this paper. I wish to focus on his fourth point given my earlier critique of "community-centric" solutions. Needham uses the term "community" in a number of different ways. It is used to describe the Salvation Army corps;[161] the whole Salvation Army;[162] the mission of the whole church;[163] and, most comprehensively, to describe the whole of creation.[164] At times Needham's use of "community" emphasizes a relational conception of the Christian life—as against an overtly individualistic personhood.

---

156. Needham, "Integrating Holiness and Community," 6.

157. Ibid.

158. Needham is noting a similar trend as identified by Ann Woodall in her term "liberal incarnationalism" with an increased reliance on social science methods and a decline in the use of theological resources.

159. Needham, "Integrating Holiness and Community," 7.

160. Ibid.

161. "faith community" on 8.

162. "an intentional Kingdom community" on 10.

163. "the community of faith" on 11.

164. "what God does in community" on 16.

However, Needham does not define the term "community" in the article and it is my contention that a lack of clarity is a point of vulnerability for contemporary Salvation Army theology and practice. Needham's lack of clarity is particularly problematic given the increasing use of "community" in reference to people outside the church whom Salvationists are called to serve. The Salvation Army has invested significantly in community development programs staffed by people with professional development qualifications who, I fear, are overly reliant on secular development theory.

Needham is certainly not recommending a secularist Salvation Army. He is reacting against an individualistic conception of holiness which leads to a "spiritualist privateness which abandons community"[165] and adopts a dualistic theology disconnecting body and soul—at the expense of the body. However, the slipperiness of the term "community" could give a reading of Needham as promoting an Anthropological Model of doing theology.[166] Bevans argues that the anthropological perspective on the goodness of "the human context is perhaps too naïve and doesn't recognize enough the sinfulness and error into which human beings can fall. There is a tendency as well to romanticize cultural practices and to forget that culture is something that is always changing as it encounters factors that challenge it and even subvert it."[167]

I have detected this tone in some of the community development and health resources produced by The Salvation Army in the past decade. I restate, this is not Needham's intention, but the word "community" needs to be handled with considerable care.

SUMMARY

This chapter has described and analyzed the culture and context of Salvation Army practice by engaging with three theologian practitioners—Wesley, Booth, and Needham. All three provide insights into how Salvation Army health ministry can better participate in God's work of restoring health to a fallen creation. Wesley's theological anthropology and eschatological *telos* are helpful in appreciating the value of health and medicine. Booth focused on the breakdown of Victorian society's

---

165. Ibid., 7–8.
166. Bevans, *An Introduction to Theology in Global Perspectives*, 174–77.
167. Ibid., 176.

relationship with the London residuum. His solution for salvation of body and soul was an institutionally based scheme run by faithful soldiers. The process of describing and analyzing the culture and context has identified a number of tensions in Salvation Army practice following the publication of *In Darkest England*.

Needham has gone some way to addressing these tensions in four key areas of Salvation Army theology and practice: ecclesiology, personhood and health, the role of institutions, and the importance of relationships in community. I seek to build on these insights and experience to assist The Salvation Army towards a more faithful future. The next chapter will engage the issues in a theological dialogue with the work of Augustine, Hauerwas, and Bretherton among others.

5

A Soteriological Orientation for Health Ministry

THEOLOGICAL RESOURCES ARE THROUGHOUT this book but Chapter 5 specifically examines the theological significance of the issues and conclusions reached to date. The aim, following Swinton and Mowatt's model of theological enquiry, is to draw out "implicit and explicit theological dimensions" and "search for authentic revelation in a spirit of critical faithfulness and chastened optimism."[1] I intend to show that Salvationists, from all parts of the world and different economic situations, share the common *telos* of "healthy persons" despite inequalities in context. This *telos* is grounded in the shared Christian faith, the common salvation story, which is lived out and sustained through shared beliefs, habits, and practices.

Scripture is a key resource in self-understanding for the community of faith called Salvationists. It is not enough to treat Scripture—and the soteriological imperative it proclaims—as merely background information buried in the footnotes of practice. Therefore, this chapter gives Scripture priority in shaping an understanding of "healthy persons" by using the overarching narrative of soteriology in the Bible—creation, fall, and redemption—to structure the discussion. This is not an isolationist move. While some secularists may object to giving sacred texts an influential role in the process of decision-making, this should not tempt FBOs to pretend the foundational resources of their faith are not significant.

---

1. Swinton and Mowat, *Practical Theology and Qualitative Research*, 96.

Two theologians inform the dialogue in this chapter and provide insights from the Bible and Christian tradition for this practical theology. Augustine's eschatology provides a framework for situating "healthy persons" within the world but not of the world. Stanley Hauerwas, originally a Methodist, offers perspectives on medicine and the Church that will be helpful in generating a faithful orientation for Salvation Army health ministry.

CREATED AS PERSONS-IN-RELATION

The starting point in developing a soteriological orientation for Salvation Army health ministry is an understanding of God and his intention in creating people. Therefore, this reflection begins by focusing on the theological concept of personhood as it is foundational for the *telos* of "healthy persons" recommended by this book as a faithful orientation for Salvation Army health ministry.

Christian theology claims to be able to speak truthfully about all present realities because "the God of Abraham is God of all the Earth, not limited in power by location, nationality or particular function."[2] Through their understanding of God, the Church, and FBOs can seek to engage with all created realities and are not confined by location, nationality, or function. In other words, the *telos* of Salvation Army health ministry is not necessarily limited by national or functional boundaries but, instead, depends on its theology. To appreciate and sustain such an orientation requires a confident articulation of "all created realities in relation to God through Jesus Christ, and the Holy Spirit, and of God to whom we are thus related."[3]

The Trinitarian nature of God is, therefore, foundational to the articulation of the *telos* of "healthy persons." John Zizioulas links the divine and human personhood in a particular fashion: "Both in the case of God and of man (sic) the identity of a person is recognized and posited clearly and unequivocally, but this is so only in and through a relationship, and not through an objective ontology in which this identity would be isolated, pointed at, and described in itself. Personal identity is totally lost if isolated, for its ontological condition is relationship."[4]

---

2. Holmes, "Introduction," x.
3. Ibid., xi.
4. Zizioulas, "On Being a Person," 46.

Our understanding of "personhood" should not be reduced to individual qualities or capacities but rather centers on "who we are" rather than "what we are." The Christian theological understanding of "who we are" is grounded in the belief that God created man and woman in his own image (Genesis 1:26). The two dimensions of divine personal being—otherness and relation—are central in appreciating the implications of persons-in-the-image of God. Being made in the image of God means being created unique (other) and "recognizing relationship as constitutive of creaturely personhood."[5]

Bretherton recognizes a threefold pattern of personhood after the example of the incarnate Jesus whereby "we are the same as all other creatures, we are more like some persons than others and we are also like no other person; each person is unique."[6] This threefold pattern of personhood is helpful in describing a pattern for "healthy persons." "Healthy persons" seek three aspects of personhood: a common humanity; a commitment to specific people; and appreciation of individual uniqueness. These three aspects of personhood need to be held in tension. An overemphasis on one aspect of the threefold pattern results in distortion of God's intention. An over emphasis on commonality can lead to an undervaluing of person and place; an over emphasis on specific location can lead to an extreme nationalism while an over emphasis on individuality leads to extreme individualism with a rejection of responsibility to anyone else. God's created intention was for "healthy persons" to have the capacity to dwell with the tension of appreciating their humanity, location and uniqueness.

There are dangers in making presumptions on the nature and personhood of people from the doctrine of God. An over-emphasis could lead to an overestimation of the capacity of persons or a reading of the nature and personhood of God conditioned by human experience.[7] The question is never how the human personality offers insight into the divine personality, but rather how "insights concerning the character of divine personhood can be creatively applied to elucidate the understanding of human personhood."[8]

---

5. Bretherton, *Christianity and Contemporary Politics*, 146.
6. Ibid., 147.
7. Rudman, *Concepts of Person and Christian Ethics*, 188.
8. Schwöbel, "Introduction," 13.

Rudman identifies two approaches to understanding the concept of human personhood rooted in an appreciation of the divine personhood: rationality and relationality.[9] These are not incompatible concepts but are complementary ways of developing a deeper understanding of "healthy persons." Rationality tends to make personhood primarily a matter of the rational qualities of soul and body whereas relationality is broader in its scope.

There is a long rationality tradition within Christian ontology of personhood understanding the human person as body and soul. It argues people have a physical body (of which the mind determines the rational response) but it is temporal—it degenerates with time, eventually experiences physical death and finally decomposes. However, there is an eternal dimension to each person, described as the soul. Rationality includes the capacity to decide and act freely allowing people to choose.

This understanding of the anthropology of body and soul is grounded in the doctrine of God and the creation account in Genesis. A view of the body-soul union rooted in the resurrection holds that the bodily person and humanity in general exist in a social and political economy, which is determined by the loving social relations of the Trinity and the intrinsically social nature of humans made in its image.[10] However, there are dangers for rationality when it is isolated from relationality.

These dangers are highlighted in Descartes' dualist conception of an intellectual mind and mechanical body. As Colin Gunton argued: "Despite Descartes attempts to show that his mind is more intimately related to his body than a pilot is to a ship, we are inescapably presented with the image of a mind pushing around a mechanical body."[11] Dualism can result in an individualistic conception of personhood, an under-appreciation of the body and the conclusion that true humanity is found in soul-life. A body-soul dualism is problematic for a Christian theology frame as there is a "far-ranging consensus of biblical exegetes that the view of what it means to be human in biblical writings has a strong holistic emphasis, depicting human beings as a unity of soul and body, mind and flesh."[12]

---

9. Rudman, *Concepts of Person and Christian Ethics*, 171.
10. Caspary, "On Health," 157.
11. Gunton, "Trinity, Ontology and Anthropology," 47.
12. Schwöbel, "Introduction," 8.

Relationality acknowledges the divine origins of "healthy persons" and argues it is only through this primal relationship that people can relate to God and each other as relational beings. "Humans bear the divine image, so that in and through their relationships, they reveal something of the Creator, as bearers of the divine image, and are called to act *in loco Dei*."[13] "Healthy persons" are therefore not defined as "individuals" but rather as "persons-in relation."

Zizioulas, from a Trinitarian perspective, argues that all personhood is communal, for it derives from the Trinitarian mystery of persons-in-communion.[14] He emphasizes the ontological reality of persons, their essential co-existence in community based on the ontology of the Trinitarian Godhead. For Zizioulas, personhood is not about any kind of capacity or quality (moral, social, or physical) but a claim to uniqueness in terms of hypostasis. Therefore, absolute uniqueness is possible only by appreciating the relationship between God and "healthy persons" which arises freely from a relationship, which is constituted by its unbrokenness. The identity of an individual person is recognized and posited clearly and unequivocally, but this is only so in and through a relationship.

However, this should not lead to a negation of each person as made in the image of God. "Healthy persons" are persons-in-relationship but not dominated by other persons. They are "not simply a passive recipient, but someone who brings herself to expression in the world."[15] "Healthy persons" have their own complex agency and motivation and are able to act on their own behalf but do so without the negation of their status as persons-in-relationship.

In summary, it is essential to appreciate all people as created in the image of God, integrated body-soul who are persons-in-relation. This fuller understanding of personhood—in contrast to early Salvation Army theology and practice highlighted in the previous chapter—is in accord with Needham's repair work and aids the recovery from a drift towards dualism. The next section begins to develop a theological understanding of the Fall.

---

13. McArdle, "The Relational Person within a Practical Theology of Health Care," 194–95.

14. Zizioulas, "Human Capacity and Human Incapacity," Zizioulas, "On Being a Person."

15. Bretherton, *Christianity and Contemporary Politics*, 146.

THE IMPLICATIONS OF THE FALL

As a consequence of the Fall, Christianity teaches that relationships are disrupted and the image of God in people is distorted. The experience of the brokenness of God's created order and the work of repair have been interlinked by theologians down the ages—therefore I do not attempt to neatly detach reflections on the Fall from reflections on redemption. However, this next section will predominately reflect on the fallen state of health and medicine while the next section focuses on the work of redemption and recovery.

The Fallen State of Health

Augustine's theological reflections on health and medicine start from an understanding of human life that integrates the natural, socio-personal, and spiritual as the sphere where the presence of God's love is intrinsic, and can be recognized and responded to.[16] At the same time, Augustine's eschatology requires recognition of limitations of the body and medicine. Augustine has little interest in the definition of disease or health but rather in its meaning. Augustine saw health as a temporal good—helpful for humans on their pilgrimage towards eternal happiness.

Drawing on Almut Caspary's work, I note Augustine did not ignore the reality of living in a fallen world. Due to the Fall, the image of God's love in humans is in need of renewal and restoration.[17] Augustine viewed suffering as a practical challenge to his faith, requiring a practical response, and argued that the restoration of health belonged to the broader narrative of salvation—the work of redemption. Augustine developed five aspects of health based on the understanding of medicine as viewed in the context of salvation cooperating with God's desire for "healthy persons."[18] Firstly, bodily health reflects the goodness of the created body. Second, it is a *particular* aspect of *general* well being; it is nothing but an interim step towards a better and more certain health, the health of the whole person. Third, both being (*that* humans exist) and well being (*how* humans exist) had their cause in God. That humans live is due to the one who created life; that they live happily, healthily, or joyfully is due to the one who causes happiness, health, or joy: to God we must attribute both

---

16. Caspary, "On Health," 16.
17. Ibid. 25.
18. Ibid. 206–8.

the being and well-being of all things. Fourth, temporal health, as well as happiness and joy, reflect eternal health and happiness, which is granted to the believer in the fullness of his or her salvation. Temporal health at the same time may be a sign of God's restoring grace already present in this world. Fifth, medicine may be an effective means of healing. Yet it is not the only means of healing: God is known to heal through (i) baptism and (ii) prayer—ways of healing which are indicative of the restoration of physical health in the order of salvation.

As noted earlier, Wesley followed the Augustinian conception of health and medicine. However, there are hints in Wesley—and strong overtones in early Salvationist writing—of a priority for "soul-health" over "body-health." Hauerwas helps to recover an Augustinian understanding and repair any dualistic reading of Wesley viewing the body as "non-matter" arguing this would not have been understood by people prior to modernity: "Accordingly our common distinction between the inner and outer, the individual and the social body, were unknown or understood quite differently. For example it was assumed by many in the ancient world that the individual human body was but an instance of the social body."[19] This is a crucial point for Hauerwas as it serves as a corrective against "the endemic individualism and rationalism that has too often been thought necessary or at least confused with a concern with holiness."[20] To be a Christian is to become a member of the body of Christ and that means interconnectivity and interdependence—we are disciples. This is difficult for contemporary Christians to appreciate but Hauerwas identifies the importance of times of sickness as a help to contemporary Christians in accepting the reality of our bodies.

Hauerwas argues not merely for a right understanding of fallenness but also the right response when confronted by the consequential and unavoidable reality of illness and suffering. Hauerwas encourages Christians to learn to be at peace with themselves and gain an ability to accept the mystery of suffering.[21] Illness is an opportunity to "discover that we are part of a story that we did not make up."[22] Such a perspective enables "healthy persons" to resist the temptation to reduce the body to a "thing"

---

19. Paraphrasing Dale Martin Hauerwas, *Sanctify Them in the Truth*, 81.
20. Ibid., 80.
21. Hauerwas and Coles, *Christianity, Democracy and the Radical Ordinary*, 313.
22. Hauerwas, *Sanctify Them in the Truth*, 84.

or something other than "me." Illness forces "healthy persons" to confront the temporal nature of the body and gives opportunity to value physical frailty in the context of eschatological hope. This is an important development in describing the orientation of "healthy persons." The removal of all suffering has never been the experience of Christians. Rather, it is the appreciation of the experience of suffering. Hauerwas notes: "The ultimate purpose and meaning behind Christian suffering in the New Testament is spiritual maturity. And the ultimate goal in spiritual maturity is a close dependence upon Christ based upon a childlike trust. Thus illness is seen as an opportunity for growth in faith and trust in God."[23]

This section of the book is theologically reflecting upon the impact of the Fall upon health, illness, and medicine. Reflecting on the writings of Augustine and Hauerwas has highlighted the dangers of Wesley and Booth's mechanistic worldview. This section has emphasized the importance of appreciating not only the purpose of health but also the importance of viewing suffering and illness as also being opportunities to serve God's purposes. In light of these important conclusions, the remainder of this section reflects on the practice of contemporary medicine in dialogue with Hauerwas.

The Fallen State of Medicine

One result of the Fall of humanity from perfect union with God has been the rise of misplaced confidence in the capacity of individuals to work out their own health and salvation. This often presents as a denial of the relational dimensions of personhood and the priority of the body over the soul (and in some cases, a complete denial of any soul-life). In recent centuries, western societies have increasingly embraced the notion of the "autonomous rational individual." To take this flawed conception to its illogical conclusion, only individual persons can have a particular moral status. Relationships are merely contractual. The individual autonomous unit is the "substance" of the human being, while relationships are simply "accidents."[24]

Hauerwas is sympathetic to the critique of modern medicine offered by Michel Foucault and others that medicine is a god that has failed. It is not only that medicine offers the fallen world an alternative soteriology;

---

23. Idem., "Why Medicine Needs the Church," 543.
24. McArdle, "The Relational Person," 239.

Hauerwas disputes the mode of liberation it professes. Medicine has become a legitimating ideology allowing some people to control others in the name of liberation. Hauerwas believes many people have accepted this critique and are in thrall to medicine. He argues: "Modern medicine was formed by a modern culture that forced upon medicine the impossible role of bandaging the wounds of societies that are built upon the premise that God does not matter. Such social orders, which we rightly call liberal, take as their central problem how to secure cooperation among self-interested individuals who have nothing in common other than their desire to survive. Cooperation is secured by bargains being struck that will presumably secure the best outcome possible for each individual."[25]

As a result, society has become "tyrannized by the agents of medicine because we have voluntarily vested them with too much power."[26] However, Hauerwas does not blame doctors and health professionals for this situation: "No one can or should be blamed. The simple fact is that we are getting precisely the kind of medicine we deserve. Modern medicine exemplifies a secular social order shaped by mechanistic economic and political arrangements, arrangements that are in turn shaped by the metaphysical presumptions that our existence has no purpose other than what we arbitrarily create."[27]

Hauerwas, in accord with Polanyi, analyzes modern medicine as an example of running of society as an adjunct to the market with the consequential loss of appreciating persons-in-relations and the promotion of commodification, instrumentalization and "autonomous rational individuals." Hauerwas notes the effect of the alliance between modern medicine and the market-state. Providing "the best medical care possible" is one of the leading claims and ambitions of the liberal state[28] but, Hauerwas contends, such an ambition "is built on the denial of its own tragic finitude."[29] The power given and claimed by medicine creates tensions with religion in suggesting medicine can operate in its own sphere separate from God's mission to heal the world. This leads medicine—including faith-based

---

25. Hauerwas, "How Christians Should Be Sick," 352.
26. Idem., "Why Medicine Needs the Church," 545.
27. Idem., "How Christians Should Be Sick," 354.
28. Hauerwas and Coles, *Christianity, Democracy and the Radical Ordinary*, 2.
29. Ibid., 3.

health services for the poorest people—to be "constantly tempted to offer a form of salvation that religiously may come close to idolatry."[30]

One example of the individualization of modern medicine is the increasing specialization of healthcare. As noted previously, there is a global trend encouraging patients to seek specialist medical care. The expectation, fed by the commercialization of health care—is that specialist doctors are better equipped to "fix" their bodies than a general practitioner. This is a flawed expectation. It results in patients being charged more to see physicians who know more and more about less and less in the expectation that these specialists will make fewer mistakes. Hauerwas notes the specialization of modern medicine "ironically results in more mistakes, since, as a matter of fact, the patient happens to be more than the sum of his parts. Unfortunately, he is increasingly cared for by a medicine that is something less than the sum of its specializations."[31]

The alternative soteriology promised by modern medicine is problematic not just for theology but also for medicine. Doctors and other health workers are expected not simply to cure but also to care—to be present in the patient's pain. Hauerwas argues this is not an easy commitment to sustain: "None of us has the resources to see too much pain without that pain's hardening us. Without such a hardening, something we sometimes call by the name of professional distance, we fear we will lose the ability to feel at all. Yet physicians cannot help but be touched and, thus, tainted by the world of the sick."[32]

Hauerwas argues the first commitment of medical personnel is to be a human presence in the face of suffering and resist the temptation towards fixing the machine. However, mere human sympathy is an inadequate resource to sustain the arduous task of presence. Hauerwas argues that modern medicine needs people of faith (and specifically the practice of the Church) to embody such a presence in their lives that has become "the marrow of their habits."

> The church claims to be such a community, a people called out by a God who is always present to us, both in our sin and in our faithfulness. Because of God's faithfulness we are supposed to be a people who have learned how to be faithful to one another by

---

30. Stanley Hauerwas, "Why Medicine Needs the Church," 544.
31. Idem., "How Christians Should Be Sick," 354.
32. Idem., "Why Medicine Needs the Church," 551.

our willingness to be present, with all our vulnerabilities, to one another. For what does our God require of us other than our unfailing presence in the midst of the world's sin and pain? Thus our willingness to be ill and to ask for help, as well as our willingness to be present with the ill is no special or extraordinary activity but a form of Christian obligation to be present to one another in and out of pain.[33]

This is a key insight for FBOs seeking to engage in health ministry for the poorest people. Rather than adopting the flawed categories of medical success developed from a perspective of liberal secular individualism, FBOs need to re-envision responses to illness based on faithful presence and other practices that enable unhealthy individuals to experience fullness of life as "healthy persons." Without such a *telos* and sustaining practices, FBOs are increasingly vulnerable to the idolatrous temptation of seeking to fix the health of the poorest people without the practice being enriched by Christian habits, practices, and resources. As argued in Chapter 2, the market-state solutions for the health of the poorest people are failing to adequately respond and it will be a tragedy if, when turned to for a solution, FBOs merely echo back the same failed solutions currently operant in secular medicine.

In summary, the discussion on the Fall has highlighted individualistic conceptions of personhood dominant in contemporary accounts of health and medicine. These are based on the illusion that the pinnacle of human existence is to be an "autonomous rational individual" with the capacity to choose and function independently of all other persons. Such an over-emphasis on the capacity of the individual tends to underplay the importance of relationships in personhood. However, there are dangers in moving too far in the other direction—from the relevant and important distinction between person and individual into an attack on individuality. The concept of "healthy persons" seeks to enhance, rather than destroy, individuality.[34]

Up to this point in Chapter 5, theologically reflecting on two aspects of the Christian story—Creation and Fall—has identified foundational soteriological concepts in the quest for a faithful *telos* for FBO health ministry. Insights from the doctrine of the Trinity, *imago Dei*, body-soul anthropology as persons-in-relations are assisting the development of a

33. Ibid., 553.
34. Rudman, *Concepts of Person and Christian Ethics*, 188.

description of "healthy persons." Health is more than physical, mental, and social but has an intrinsically spiritual dimension—rather than the temporary, individualistic conceptions underpinning much of secular medicine.

The *telos* of "healthy persons" describes people as made in the image of God, unique individuals yet in relationship with each other, who each seek the restoration of the unity of body-soul in the process of building deeper relationships with other unique "healthy persons" enabled by the grace of the triune God. Keeping body and soul together reduce the dangers of developing dual and fragmentary conceptions of human health. Faith-based health ministry orientated towards "healthy persons" is able to compare, assess, and faithfully respond to fragmented and contradictory "solutions" for good health. In light of these conclusions, the theological reflection now focuses on the theme of redemption to articulate how "healthy persons" can be faithfully present in the world.

REDEEMING "HEALTHY PERSONS"

Chapter 4 identified a number of tensions in Salvation Army practice that require attention. The creation and fall sections of this chapter have articulated a theologically informed account of anthropology and the nature of the fallen health and medicine. This has been helpful in beginning to address some of these tensions. However, the central argument throughout this book has been that attention to *telos* is key for people and organizations of faith. This section develops a fuller appreciation of the *telos* of redeeming "healthy persons" and its outworking in practice—aspects foundational to this book.

Bretherton questions MacIntyre's teleology in terms of creation and redemption. Against MacIntyre's creation-based teleology, Bretherton argues for an eschatological *telos* that affirms the created independence of nature and the ordering of nature to certain ends. Bretherton argues, these ends find their resolution and perfection in the *eschaton* and not in creation. The fulfillment of these ends is only possible insofar as they participate, through the Spirit, in the new creation inaugurated by Christ's resurrection and ascension. After the Fall, the true direction of creation's teleology is re-established in Christ. That which does not participate in Christ has a "misdirected progress" and can in "no way fulfill itself out of its own resources."³⁵ Therefore, for this book, the contribution of redemption and eschatology is central.

It is not only important to be clear about orientation and aspiration, it is also essential to appreciate current realities. The ways in which the current realities of market, state, and community influence the health of the poorest people were described and analyzed in chapters 2 and 3. This section seeks to theologically reflect on the contemporary challenges of redeeming "healthy persons" in the crowded and contested space dominated by the market-state. Augustine offers a way of conceptualizing a faithful response to the forces of market, state, and community.³⁶

As with Augustine's fifth century church, the twenty-first century church—and the part called The Salvation Army—lives in the in-between times, the *saeculum*. Christ has lived, died, risen, and ascended, but he has not yet returned. Augustine conceives of two spatial realms—the city of God, the new Jerusalem, and the earthly city, Babylon³⁷—coexisting in a single time, the *saeculum* where the citizens of each city live together until Christ returns.³⁸ Bretherton summarizes: "Citizens of both cities seek peace; however, in the earthly city peace is achieved through the imposition of one's will by the exercise of force and is at once costly in its creation, lacking in real justice and unstable in its existence."³⁹ Augustine characterizes the divisions "not as a division within society but as a division between societies."⁴⁰ Bretherton comments: "Within this framework human history is "secular" (rather than neutral): that is, it neither promises nor sets at risk the kingdom of God. The kingdom of God is established, if not fully manifest, and the "end" of history is already achieved and fulfilled in Christ. Thus the church can reside in this age, regarding its structures and pattern of life as relativized by what is to come and therefore sees them as contingent and provisional. Charles Mathewes

---

35. Bretherton, *Hospitality as Holiness*, 81.
36. Idem., *Christianity and Contemporary Politics*, 3.
37. Augustine, *The City of God*, XIV, 28.
38. Ibid., XIX, 17.
39. Bretherton, *Christianity and Contemporary Politics*, 3.
40. Ibid.

draws out the implication of this as follows: "Christians' attitude to history should not be one of anxious grasping after control, but of a relaxed playfulness."[41]

Augustine linked his conception of the two cities to the letter written by Jeremiah to the Israelites taken into exile from Jerusalem to Babylon.[42] Jeremiah assured his readers they had not been abandoned. Rather, exile was the place where God was at work and the place where they were called to work. Jeremiah writes:

> This is what the Lord Almighty, the God of Israel, says to all those I carried into exile from Jerusalem to Babylon: "Build houses and settle down; plant gardens and eat what they produce. Marry and have sons and daughters; find wives for your sons and give your daughters in marriage, so that they too may have sons and daughters. Increase in number there; do not decrease. Also, seek the peace and prosperity of the city to which I have carried you into exile. Pray to the Lord for it, because if it prospers, you too will prosper."[43]

This passage of Scripture encourages people of faith to work for the health of "Babylon," even though they wish they were in "Jerusalem." Despite the people being in exile, God's purposes were being served by the Babylonian invasion. God required them to be different—not "defensive against, isolated from, or absorbed into the dominant culture, but to be faithfully present within it."[44] God was calling his people to maintain their distinctiveness but in ways that served the common good. This is the calling to faithful presence being promoted in this book for FBOs. Hunter summarizes:

> Against the dominant liberal modernist notion that the public sphere is constituted by a diversity of autonomous and unencumbered individuals, in this view there is recognition that public diversity—whose focal metaphor is the city—is also defined collectively by multiple traditions and communities. Needless to say, some of these are very different from, if not hostile to, the community of Christian believers. But even when there is disagreement, tension, and conflict, there is also a recognition that there

---

41. Ibid., 82.
42. Augustine, *The City of God*, XIX, 26.
43. Jer 29:4–7, *New International Version*.
44. Hunter, *To Change the World*, 277.

are common goods that communities of Christians drawing on the resources of their tradition, must still hold up, pursue, work at, foster, and practice.[45]

The first section of this theological reflection on the theme of redemption has described an Augustinian theological framework. This reveals an understanding of the contemporary Christian church to be living during the time of the *saeculum*—between the time of Christ's ascension and return. The church is, therefore, a combination of the earthly city and the city of God and will be separated only at the last judgment. The church is called to be faithfully present in this place of tension and resist being instrumentalized by the state, commodified by the state or manipulated by powerful individuals within the community.

Unlike Augustine's conception of the Christian living in the *saeculum* and serving two cities, William Booth contrasts the two worlds—the present and the future, pre and post the Millennium. However, I contend, Augustine's conception of the two cities is a more theologically resilient and faithful motivation for Salvationist engagements in the world than a post-millennial construction. A revised eschatological *telos* for Salvation Army health ministry, based on an Augustinian framework retains the sense of urgency that drove The Salvation Army forward towards hope of a better world. For Booth, like Jeremiah, the people of the new Jerusalem (Salvationists) were called by God to befriend and serve Babylon, by building houses (institutions), planting gardens (farms and colonies), seeking the peace and prosperity of the exile city (emigration and colonialism).[46] Booth believed the sanctified character of the Salvationists living in the Victorian world—but orientated by the post-millennial vision—would be so attractive and compelling that the world would be changed.

Therefore, I suggest, the eschatological *telos* of "healthy persons" helps The Salvation Army move on from the post-millennial theology of William Booth. Despite the limitations of Booth's eschatology, it transformed the lives of many people by giving hope and motivation. Salvationists, eschatologically orientated and sustained by the habitual practice of Spirit-filled worship, have been faithfully presence in the world for more than 120 years. Their eschatological *telos* has been key in preventing Salvation Army ministry from succumbing to the forces of

---

45. Ibid., 279.
46. Jer 29:4–7, *New International Version*.

isomorphism and enabled more sustain faithful participation. However, an understanding of faithful presence based on Jeremiah 29 offers a more resilient narrative for twenty-first century health ministry. It offers Christian health ministry "a dynamic movement via differentiation and development through history, to an eschatological fulfillment of creation."[47]

RECOVERING INSTITUTIONS AS SERVANTS OF HEALTH AND HOLINESS

This chapter is attempting a theological reflection to enhance Salvation Army health ministry for the poorest people. To this point, there has been a theologically informed description of personhood, a critique of contemporary views on health and medicine and a reflection on the redemption opportunities for "healthy persons" as faithfully present in the world. This section will now examine two key ways in which Christian health ministry can participate in this dynamic movement through faithfully present medicine and faithfully present institutions.

One of the issues prompting this research was a need to envision a faithful role for the institutions of clinic-hospitals and congregations for the task of improving the health of the poorest people. As discussed earlier, I am proposing to recover a role for faith-based institutions against the de-institutional tendencies of FBOs and denominations in recent years. Institutions such as churches, faith-based clinic-hospitals, and schools, can play a vital role in the process of mediation between individuals, the state, and the market. Without such institutions, people struggle to be in dialogue, free from government or commercial imperatives. Such spaces are essential if people are to have the space and time to listen to each other and develop mutual trust.[48] This section will theologically reflect on the contribution of institutions and recommend the church and faith-based clinic-hospitals as institutions of healing—an alternative *polis* to the market-state, the "community," and the Third Sector. Hauerwas has developed a robust and extensive advocacy of the importance of the church as alternative *polis* and this section will build on his arguments in recovering the institutions of church and faith-based clinic-hospitals.

---

47. Bretherton, *Christianity and Contemporary Politics*, 210.
48. Idem., "A Postsecular Politics?," 19.

The Institution of Church

Hauerwas takes a position against those who think the church gains relevance or acts responsibly when it forms alliances with political, cultural, and other forces that result in the Christian *telos* and gospel becoming invisible in practice.[49] Hauerwas insists the Christian Church should concentrate on thinking and living out its own story, instead of wasting time merely repeating in religious tones the moral platitudes the world already takes for granted. Hauerwas really believes the Church has news about the human and public good to proclaim to secularist liberals[50] and, he argues, the way to best experience health and life is through the Church:

> The primary social task of the church is to be itself—that is a people who have been formed by a story that provides them with the skills for negotiating the danger of their existence, trusting in God's promise of redemption . . . Christian social ethics can only be done from the perspective of those who do not seek to control national or world history but as content to "live out of control." The church does not exist to provide an ethos for democracy or any other form of social organization, but stands as a political alternative to every nation, witnessing to the kind of social life possible for those that have been formed by the story of Christ.[51]

Therefore, the church is not incidental to the world's salvation but, based on Augustinian theology, Hauerwas argues that only politics formed by the truth of the church can claim to be truthful: "Augustine does not assume such a claim requires Christians to develop an ethic for everyone as the basis of which we might be able to determine the 'best form of government.' Rather than engage in such grand projects, the church's main task is to be what we are—God's salvation. I suspect we will do that best when we are free from the presumption that the only way to survive is to try to accept the world's way of rule on its own terms."[52]

Hauerwas is suspicious of the state, which he views as collaborating with other social realities that require menace in order to maintain power.[53] When Christianity was adopted as the state religion at the

---

49. Biggar, "Is Stanley Hauerwas Sectarian?," 143.
50. Ibid.
51. Hauerwas, *A Community of Character*, 10–11.
52. Idem., *After Christendom?*, 43.
53. Reno, "Stanley Hauerwas," 310.

time of Emperor Constantine, the Church was captured by worldly vanity and illusions of social significance. Hauerwas adopts the term "Constantinianism" to describe the ongoing conflict between the message and priorities of the Church against the worldly powers with different agendas. The result of this conflict is the Church has become "innocuous" and "weightless."[54]

The cause of the "weightless" church is any attempt to make Christianity intelligible without that set of habits called the church. For Hauerwas, the key set of habits that sustain the church is worship.

> We do not believe in God, become humble and then learn to pray, but in learning to pray we humbly discover we cannot do other than believe in God. But, of course, to learn to pray requires we learn to pray with other Christians. It means we must learn the disciplines necessary to worship God. Worship, at least for Christians, is the activity to which all our skills are ordered. That is why there can be no separation of Christian morality from Christian worship. As Christians, our worship is our morality for it is in worship we find ourselves engrafted into the story of God. It is in worship that we acquire the skills to acknowledge who we are—sinners.[55]

Hauerwas argues for the distinction between church and world not to be conceived as between realms of reality, orders of creation, and redemption or nature and supernature but rather between: "the basic personal postures of men and women, some of whom confess and others of whom do not confess that Jesus is Lord. The distinction between the church and the world is not something that God has imposed upon the world by a prior metaphysical definition, nor is it only something which timid or pharisaical Christians have built up around themselves. It is all of that in creation that has taken the freedom not yet to believe."[56]

Hauerwas's ecclesial emphasis has been criticized for the priority given to God working through the church at the expense of God's capacity to act outside of the church. This, critics fear, tends toward a sectarian position of withdrawal from the world. Fergusson writes: "I am deeply skeptical about strategies, which enthusiastically deconstruct all forms of moral consciousness, while making the strongest realist claims possible for the moral perception within the church. Apart from the intrinsic

---

54. Ibid.
55. Hauerwas, *After Christendom?*, 108.
56. Idem., "The Servant Community," 375.

implausibility of this position—can one subscribe to arguments, which seek to undermine all forms of moral realism while claiming immunity to one's own particular form?—it is at odds with much of what Christian theology has historically tried to articulate in terms of natural law, common grace, and orders of creation."[57]

Fergusson argues the central theme of Christian theology is to "determine how the will of God may be done beyond the walls of the church."[58] This criticism of Hauerwas is important. It should not diminish the distinctiveness of the church, but "when the work of the Spirit is appreciated in all spheres of life it enables the church to recognize common moral ground in making common cause with other forces, agencies, and movements—even in the absence of common moral theory."[59] Fergusson's critique highlights the importance of the church not resorting to sectarian or isolationist tendencies. The capacity to recognize "common ground" and make common cause should be a priority for all people of faith and the institutions they serve in seeking better health for the poorest people.

James Davison Hunter goes further in his criticism of the sectarian tone of Hauerwas's writing. In a recent assessment of Christianity in America, Hunter argues the "Neo-Anabaptist vision"—as he categorizes the work of Yoder, Hauerwas, McClendon, Cavanaugh, Milbank, and several others[60]—is not merely sectarian but indulges in unnecessary negativity.

> In effect, theirs is a world-hating theology. It is not impossible but it is rare, all the same, to find among any of its most prominent theologians or its popularizers, any affirmation of good in the social world and any acknowledgment of beauty in creation or truth shared in common with those outside of the church. Rare too are expressions in their public discourse of delight, joy, or pleasure with anything in creation. Their targets are different from those of the Christian Right, but their dominant witness is also a witness of negation and their language can be as hard and aggressive as that of the Christian Right. Thus, they offer little alternative to the world they critique except the existence of the church itself.[61]

57. Fergusson, *Community, Liberalism and Christian Ethics*, 7.
58. Ibid., xi.
59. Ibid.
60. Hunter, *To Change the World*, 152.
61. Ibid., 174.

While Hunter overstates his critique of the Neo-Anabaptists,[62] nevertheless, there is an over-sharp division between the church and the world in Hauerwas's work. It has been attributed to a lack of a properly articulated pneumatological eschatology.[63] His emphasis on the work of God in and through the practices of the Church has resulted in an under-emphasis on the work of the Holy Spirit in the world and outside of the church. Wells argued, a decade ago, Hauerwas needed to pay greater attention to pneumatology "lest Christians be paralyzed in their membership of other communities beside the Christian one. If the Church genuinely intends to remain committed to communities other than itself, it must be because it believes that there too God lives and reigns and it wants to be where God is, with the people he has made for his service."[64]

It is an exaggeration to argue Hauerwas is promoting a "world hating" theology. I have shown his links to Augustinian and Wesleyan theology in proposing a vision of Christian hope and health as worship-centric and relationally based. For Hauerwas, like Augustine and Wesley, to be a holy person is being able to accept forgiveness for sins and join with others who have accepted this gift and worship God worthily. None of these theologians advocates a pure individualistic conception of holiness or a withdrawal from the world. However, Hauerwas does give rightful priority to the worshipping practices of the community of faith. He writes, "As Augustine argues in *The City of God*, nothing is more important for a society than to worship God justly. Without such worship, terrible sacrifices will be made to false gods."[65]

Both worship and world-engagement are essential for people of faith. As Brian Brock argues: "Worship is not a choice about how to spend time outside of the public life of work"[66] rather "worship transforms human work into so many forms of hospitality because it attunes us to Christ in the neighbor, with his or her very material needs."[67] This is a particularly important point for Salvation Army health ministry—hospital and congregation. It is a false dichotomy to conceive of worship and the world

62. Later in his book, Hunter promotes the practice of "faithful presence" adopting the same theological arguments as the Neo-Anabaptists.
63. Bretherton, *Hospitality as Holiness*, 106.
64. Wells, *Transforming Fate into Destiny*, 98.
65. Hauerwas, *Sanctify Them in the Truth*, 11.
66. Brock, *Christian Ethics in a Technological Age*, 300.
67. Ibid., 301.

as different. Brock promotes engagement with the world on the basis of "encounter" as means of allowing "the church's way of being to rub off on secular society" as against an over-emphasis on "counter politics."[68] This opens up the opportunity for the church to not merely resist the forces of institutional isomorphism—from a position of defensiveness—but to "percolate out into the secular political consciousness."[69] The faith-based difference is, Brock argues, discovered in the "practical exploration of the political conceptualizations to which it has been directed by revelation."[70] Health ministry offers such an opportunity for practical exploration directed by theological revelation.

Therefore, in seeking healthy institutions for faith-based health ministry, two facts need to be held in tension. The church is an institution that requires attention for the worship of God, the formation and sustaining of the worshipping community of believers and as a witness to the world. At the same time, God does not abandon the creation outside of the church because of its fallen nature but, rather, through the work of the Holy Spirit is "present, active, and faithful to creatures beyond the domain of the church."[71] Through this tension, Christians can engage in health ministry (and other secular forms of employment) supported and sustained by the practices of the worshipping church. In effect, this calls for FBOs to engage in the *saeculum* as an intermediary organization—serving the interests of the earthly city of Babylon but sustained and orientated by the city of God, the new Jerusalem. As Karl Barth noted, referenced in Fergusson, it is not the uniqueness of the church that is decisive, but the uniqueness of God's self-revelation in Jesus Christ. Therefore, it is possible to witness outside of the church although the validity of the witness "must be tested by reference to Scripture, the theological traditions of the church and its impact for the life of the Christian community in the world."[72] The calling for individual disciples of Jesus is not simply a changed self-understanding but becoming "part of a different community with different set of practices."[73] This is an important point for this book

---

68. Ibid., 245.
69. Ibid.
70. Ibid., 246.
71. Fergusson, *Community, Liberalism and Christian Ethics*, 162.
72. Ibid., 2.
73. Hauerwas, *After Christendom?*, 107.

in the quest to keep faith in faith-based organizations. The *telos* is not to be sustained by individuals but rather by a different community with a different set of practices.

Hauerwas's ecclesiological convictions appear to have resulted in an overconfident assessment of the capacity of the contemporary church to build and sustain a witness of faithful presence. A more faithful (and realistic) position is to acknowledge the fragile character of Christians, the vulnerability of the church but also the transformational power of the Spirit. The Church operates in the *saeculum*—the "now" and the "not yet." The experience of "perfection" is available to the church and its members; but "not yet" has the *eschaton* been realized and the fallen world totally redeemed. Hauerwas's overconfidence in the capacity of the church in the *saeculum* is, perhaps, indicative of a North American perspective where the church has a long historical legacy, significant cultural acceptance, and is more receptive to a bullish, church-centric response against the rise of secularism. Few Christians in South Asia, East Asia, and Europe belong to such confident, culturally accepted churches. Hauerwas helpfully offers minority Christian congregations a confident ecclesiology but, perhaps, they have something to teach Hauerwas about the wisdom, humility, patience and grace needed to sustain faithful presence in the *saeculum* amid the forces of nationalist Hinduism (in parts of India), radical Islam (many parts of the world), and secularism (parts of Europe). In particular, the church and the world need intermediary institutions that serve "Babylon" but remain faithful, orientated, and sustained by "Jerusalem."

The Hospitable Hospital

During visits to Indonesia, Salvation Army leaders serving in Christian minority contexts helped me understand the value of intermediary institutions such as clinic-hospitals in serving hostile communities and building faithful relationships. The worshipping, evangelical Christian church can be perceived as confrontational, but people of all faiths usually welcome FBOs who care for the health of the poorest people without discrimination.

Hauerwas criticizes churches for being diverted from their primary task of worship and the moral formation of the community by involvement in service delivery.[74] He is also critical of church-state partner-

---

74. Ibid., 95.

ships—and, by implication, much of The Salvation Army's health ministry for the poorest people as it is funded directly or indirectly by government agencies. The risks of isomorphism are acknowledged throughout this book but Hauerwas's resistance to church-state partnerships needs to be challenged in light of the health needs of the poorest people, the cost of funding a faith-based health ministry—unaffordable without some form of subsidy—and the value of faithfully orientated health ministry. Despite the risks, the church, the state, and the people benefit from discovering and then seeking a faithful understanding of health sustained by institutions of church and faith-based clinic-hospital with the potential to build bridges into hostile, unhealthy communities, and resist the forces of the market. For this end, I contend, state funding can be accepted.

Having acknowledged the need for FBOs to engage in partnerships, particularly with hospitals, Hauerwas's warnings must be taken seriously. Hospitals will only sustain faithful characteristics if attention is given to creating and sustaining their character. Central to the task of faithfully orientating health institutions and promoting faithful practice is the contribution of "presence." Hauerwas argues:

> Unless there is a body of people who have learned the skills of presence, the world of the ill cannot help but become a separate world both for the ill and for those who care for them. Only a community that is pledged not to fear the stranger—and illness always makes us a stranger to ourselves and others—can welcome the continued presence of the ill in our midst. The hospital is, after all, first and foremost a house of hospitality along the way of our journey with finitude. It is our sign that we will not abandon those who have become ill simply because they currently are suffering the sign of that finitude. If the hospital, as too often is the case today, becomes but a means of isolating the ill from the rest of us, then we have betrayed its central purpose and distorted our community and ourselves.[75]

Hauerwas's conception of the hospital as a "house of hospitality," where the "skill of presence" is sustained and taught, brings together the character of hospitality with the institution of hospital. This is an important emphasis for two reasons. Firstly, it brings the congregation into contact with suffering. This counters the trend of separating off the sick to be "fixed" by the professionals. The church can always learn from

---

75. Idem., "Why Medicine Needs the Church," 554.

the experience of suffering and should not run away from it. Secondly, bringing people of faith into the hospital offers the opportunity for the health professionals to access the skills and resources necessary to relate deeply to sick and suffering people. In contrast, the dominant biomedical model of health care has a tendency for health professionals to become distanced from suffering by the institutional protection of hospital walls and professional codes of conduct. Hauerwas argues that medicine needs the church not as a reference point for "morality" but as "a resource of the habits and practices necessary to sustain the care of those in pain over the long term. For it is no easy matter to be with the ill, especially when we cannot do much for them other than simply be present."[76]

There is a long Christian witness to the value and importance of health ministry characterized by hospitality. St Benedict is quoted as saying, "Care for the sick must rank above and before all else, so that they may truly be served as Christ."[77] Likewise, John Wesley prioritized the importance of health ministry. In his journal entry for 24 November 1760, Wesley noted the dual benefits of visiting the sick for the Methodists: "I visited as many as I could of the sick . . . and that both for our own sake and theirs. For theirs, as it is so much more comfortable to them, and as may then assist them in spirituals as well as temporals. And for our own, as it is far more apt to soften our heart and to make us naturally care for each other."[78]

Health ministry enables people of faith to be present in the world's suffering. Hospitality is the social practice that best embodies and witnesses to the nature of the relationship between Christians and non-Christians. It is a social practice with a long track record of shaping relations between the church and its neighbors. Through diverse initiatives the church hosts "the life together of its neighbors and enables that life to bear witness to its eschatological possibilities."[79] Bretherton envisions hospitality as an "eschatological social practice" which is "inspired and empowered by the Holy Spirit, who enables the church to host the life of its neighbors without the church being assimilated to, or colonized by,

---

76. Ibid., 553.
77. Benedict, *The Rule of St. Benedict*, 38.
78. Webster, "Health of Soul and Health of Body," 216.
79. Bretherton, *Hospitality as Holiness*, 196.

or having to withdraw from, the life of its neighbors."[80] The benefits of the practice of hospitality are substantial when it

> is a way of countering patronizing or excluding relations between strangers because it demands that the hosts become de-centered and transform their understanding of themselves in order both to make room for and to encounter the other ... Second, hospitality refuses the fantasy of neutral ground on which all may meet as equals: all places are already filled by one tradition or another ... Hospitality is a way of framing how such mutual ground can be forged in a context where the space—be it geographic, cultural, or political—is already occupied and no neutral, uncontested place is available. To be hospitable is not simply to accommodate another, but, on a Christian account at least, it involves a process of re-configuring wherein both oneself and the other change in order that all may encounter God and each other in new ways.[81]

By being attentive to the characteristics of hospitality, FBOs can serve as intermediaries between the worshipping community of the church and the health concerns of people of other faiths. There is no necessary conflict between the commitments Christians have in and to the church and their commitment to improving the health of the poorest people. However, the faithful response required of FBOs to achieve real encounter, dialogue, and understanding is not by seeking out some lowest common denominator of general belief shared by all. The characteristic of faithful hospitality is developed and sustained when church and clinic-hospital pay attention to habits and practices intrinsic to the Christian tradition.

Placing Limits on Hospitals

This book notes how the bio-medical approach is a market-centric "solution" that is increasingly dominating—and damaging—health services around the world. The bio-medical model—which unavoidably leads to hospital-centrism—emphasizes the "fixing" role of health services (advocating for more technologically complex drugs and curative treatments, in specialist hospitals by doctors with specialist qualifications) rather than prioritizing a relational approach to health care. A relational approach to health emphasizes a holistic appreciation of "healthy persons"

---

80. Ibid., 188.
81. Idem., "A Postsecular Politics?," 13.

and engages with the totality of health (physical, emotional, spiritual, and mental) through integrated primary health initiatives including prevention, education, treatment, and care activities. The involvement of people of faith, not just in the hospital building but being present at every link of an integrated chain of care from-home-to-hospital-and-back, is a richer, more faithfully present description of hospitable, health ministry than the bio-medical model.

By envisioning a wider role for faith-based health care beyond the hospital and biomedical framework, "ordinary" people can be involved in health ministry. Under the bio-medical framework, health work is left to the professionally trained. However, there are many skills required for health and healing that the bio-medical establishment are unable or unwilling to offer. For example, one of the key skills in the practice of hospitality is listening. The ability to hear (in all the multiple dimensions inferred by the word) is key in the process of getting to know each other and understanding oneself. It is not possible to know another person without the ability to listen. With poor listening unhealthy people—particularly poor people—are reduced to an instrument or a commodity.[82]

If churches, clinic-hospitals, and other FBOs seek the characteristics of hospitality—such as deep listening—and are able to work together with the wider community for the common good a "real encounter, dialogue, and understanding can be generated as a by-product of shared civic action."[83] A hospital or place of worship may be a starting point for such a venture but the work of community-based primary health care also offers a valuable space for meaningful dialogue. Through the process of working together on tasks that achieve a common good, social relations are developed between people with different perspectives and faith. It is evidenced by a "common action that is a negotiated, multi-lateral endeavor."[84] This is the basis for establishing "mutual interest."

It is my contention that if faith-based health institutions are to retain a focus on developing congregation and community-based PHC initiatives, they must not become too large or else they will become a distraction. The biomedical model continually pushes towards expansion, greater specialization, and technologization of medicine. As a consequence, the

82. For a fuller treatment of the importance of listening as faithful witness see Idem., *Christianity and Contemporary Politics*, 99–104.

83. Idem., "A Postsecular Politics?," 11.

84. Ibid., 14.

A Soteriological Orientation for Health Ministry   151

treatment aspects of health ministry are prioritized above the primary health care priorities of care, education, and prevention. Such distractions and diversions have led some influential voices in faith-based health ministry to recommend the Church withdraw from all treatment provision and limit its role to care, education, and prevention activities.[85] This position is often justified on the grounds that it is the state's responsibility to provide health care for its people and FBOs should not allow government to avoid its responsibilities. Although people of faith should advocate governments to care for its most vulnerable citizens, those recommending the closure of faith-based clinic-hospitals (whose main function is treatment), appear naïve in presuming the withdrawal of the faith-based treatment facilities will somehow spur the market-state into action. There is no evidence to support this optimism.

If funding for FBO health initiatives to improve the health of the poorest people and to care for them while ill continues to drift towards non-treatment, non-institution, non-church approaches, the church will be abdicating its God-given responsibility for the sickest, most vulnerable, poorest people in the world to state or market providers. This cannot be a faithful response to the health of the poorest people. Therefore, this book argues the church should encourage the state to partner with faith-based intermediary groups such as clinic-hospital-based health services. Creative partnerships with state and/or market providers will be unavoidable. Such partnerships can be formed on the basis of "mutual interest" but require a "civilized culture of conflict" informed and sustained by the theological resources of the church.

However, this leaves FBOs in an uncomfortable place—a location of "tension-dwelling." In a recent work, Hauerwas argues this is the right place for Christians to inhabit:

> Jesus lets the world truly be the world by refiguring our very sense of topography, such that the edge-effect . . . becomes the metaphor not just for the possible meeting ground between different communities, but, more importantly, for the character of generative life-giving places and modes of dwelling as such. In this sense, vulnerable edges are seen to run throughout different communities and landscapes in ways that—insofar as we live them vulnerably,

---

85. Staff from BN, the Norwegian church agency who manage the dispersal of Norwegian state funds to faith-based development and health projects, made this argument to me in 2008.

which is at once our only possibility for living well and often a genuine danger—"are not predictable." It is the vulnerably undulating unpredictable landscape that is a constitutive dimension of the world into which Jesus (and radical democracy) would call us to recognize and work.[86]

One way of living with the vulnerability for the church (and FBOs)—I suggest—is to partner with those who do not share the same *telos* but are willing to work in a mutual spirit of hospitality for the betterment of the poorest and most vulnerable people. Health ministry provides opportunities for generous involvement and for the "church to be the church" by showing the world that it is the world, but this does not mean the church and the world cannot partner together for the common good. As Bretherton notes, "the link between Christianity and democracy is best understood as an exploratory and mutually disciplined partnership."[87] Without partnerships with the nation-state—even if dictators rather than democrats lead the nation—the church will withdraw from health ministry because it is too difficult for a fragile church. However, such a withdrawal will leave the church—and the people it serves—more vulnerable and fragile. Therefore, health ministry to the poorest people who live in countries characterized by completely dysfunctional nation-states is a creative and necessary place for the church—and FBOs seeking to be intermediary organizations—to inhabit.

SUMMARY

This chapter has developed a soteriological description for health ministry using a narrative theology framework to develop a description of the *telos* of "healthy persons" and a means to enable the development of such "healthy persons." The soteriological framework of creation, fall, and redemption structured an engagement with a number of theologians including Augustine, Hauerwas, and Bretherton. The chapter critiqued the conception of people as "autonomous rational individuals" and suggested that FBOs should be orientated towards the account of "healthy persons" who are redeemed through the work of Jesus Christ, empowered by the Holy Spirit, and sustained by the habits and practices of the Church.

---

86. Hauerwas and Coles, *Christianity, Democracy and the Radical Ordinary*, 15.
87. Bretherton, *Christianity and Contemporary Politics*, 105.

The individualistic biomedical framework underpinning contemporary medical practice has been critiqued in dialogue with Hauerwas's analysis of contemporary medical practice. The eschatological *telos* proposed for FBOs is not merely sustained by well-meaning individuals but rather by the habits and practices of the congregation. This position appreciates the work of the Holy Spirit—within and beyond the church—as a means of Christian health ministry transforming social relations—and the health of the poorest people—in partnership with people who have a different *telos*.

Finally, the chapter theologically reflected on the contribution of the institution of clinic-hospital and congregation in improving the health of the poorest people. The church is to be appreciated as an alternate *polis* and place for worship, formation, and witness to an unbelieving world. Similarly, the recovery of the institution of clinic-hospital as a support to community-based primary health initiatives was promoted. Such faith-based institutions, I argue, can be intermediary organization working for the good of Babylon while remaining teleologically faithful and sustained by the city of God. It is not easy, but it is possible, to sustain such an orientation by institutions despite the pressure to comply with the commodification and instrumental agendas of the market-state.

6

Formulating Revised Forms of Practice

THIS BOOK SET OUT to answer a question: "What characterizes faithfully orientated Salvation Army health ministry in the twenty-first century?" The answer, I propose, is for Salvation Army health ministries to promote and present opportunities for people to enjoy life as "healthy persons"; people whose lives are soteriologically orientated and characterized by their relationship with God and are faithfully present in the world. This *telos* of "healthy persons" transcends geographical, economic, and racial boundaries.

    This final chapter draws together the characteristics of faithfully orientated Salvation Army health ministry and makes recommendations for further *recovery* of faithfulness. The word *recovery* is associated with healing and is preferred to the mechanistic overtones in the language of repair. The language of recovery and healing is important in the overall task of reorientating practice towards a more faithful eschatological *telos*. My recommendations are not limited to Salvation Army health ministry—that would fall into the trap of understanding "health" as simply a biomedical construction. A pursuit after the telos of "healthy persons" is an appropriate *telos* for all Salvationists, employees, volunteers, and others who seeking to be "faithfully present," participating in God's work of redeeming the world. This chapter will complete the fourth and final stage of the practical theology framework: formulating revised forms of practice.[1]

The question driving this book and the answers generated are unashamedly faith-tradition specific as I am seeking to respond to the circumstances challenging The Salvation Army. However, I believe that this book, and the practical theology model of enquiry it demonstrates, can be of assistance to people from other faith traditions as they explore what it means for them to be faithfully present in the world.

MOVEMENT

The first characteristic of faithfully present Salvation Army health ministry is *movement*. The early Salvationists—like the Methodists before them and the Pentecostals after them—believed their new expression of Christianity was the dynamic work of God. The Booths insisted on calling The Salvation Army a *movement* and not a church—as noted in chapter 4 based on an understanding of The Salvation Army as a new work of God distinct from the Church and a means for God inaugurating the new Kingdom.

By proposing the characteristic of movement, I am not proposing a return for The Salvation Army to the ecclesial wilderness. Rather, I envision a flexible, agile, ambitious Salvation Army movement, part of the wider Christian Church, modeling a relevant, faithful, twenty-first century tension-dwelling engagement in difficult situations resulting in an improvement in the health of the poorest people. This is not a new idea for The Salvation Army. In the late nineteenth and early twentieth century, Salvationists embarked upon a wide range of initiatives as they sought to win the world for God. They embraced new ways of working with dynamic creativity. Sir Winston Churchill, former British Prime Minister, is credited with quipping after witnessing Salvation Army work during World War Two, "Where there's a need there's The Salvation Army." Churchill summed up the confidence and diversity of Salvation Army mission, identity, and presence around the world in the toughest places. A consequence of the Churchillian quip was Salvationists began using it as a public relation slogan resulting in justifying an ever increasing and diverse range of social services. Such diversity carries with it the

---

1. Swinton and Mowat, *Practical Theology and Qualitative Research*, 96.

risks of losing mission focus resulting in dilution, diversion, and a hollowing out of Christian identity.

Although this book has noted some evidence of loss of faithfulness, The Salvation Army's multifaceted identity also offers invaluable opportunities to be faithfully present. A faithfully orientated *movement* with a multifaceted-identity can be advantageous in places where relationships need developing, trust has to be established, and hospitality offered particularly to people with a different faith or worldview. Working to improve the health of the poorest people is an example of the benefits of a multifaceted identity. As argued earlier, identity and location should not have priority over orientation. Therefore, Salvation Army health ministry characterized by *movement* and seeking after an eschatological *telos* of "healthy persons" can be faithfully present in the world in a variety of contextually appropriate guises.

However, care is required in the use of guise. The military metaphor offers significant benefits in terms of identity, visibility, adaptability, and responsiveness. Unfortunately, the adoption of civil service bureaucratic systems into The Salvation Army can allow a mechanistic, structural mindset[2] to become more influential than the characteristics of a *movement*. This problem of mechanistic managerialism is not limited to The Salvation Army. Brian Brock notes the rise of "rational management into every corner of modern political relations including that of the churches" and warns against the imposition of a "mechanistic, army-like manner" on the life of the church.[3]

In the period since 1878, when William Booth and his followers started using the name The Salvation Army and adopted military terminology, there has been a tension between the characteristic of *movement* and those of mechanistic managerialism. Salvationists remembering their long tradition of reliance on the Holy Spirit are often quick to confront leaders or managers who are promoting anything with restrictive mechanistic tendencies. This appreciation of pneumatological eschatology has been a corrective to the managerialists and a source of inspiration to those promoting the characteristics of movement. A pneumatological eschatology enables the contribution of people of faith to be appreciated as participants in God's work of healing the world. The characteristics of

---

2. A similar argument was made by Needham, *Community in Mission*, 48–51.
3. Brock, *Christian Ethics in a Technological Age*, 238.

movement—flexible, agile, and alert in the power of the Spirit—are particularly valuable when confronted by the market and state's tendency to close down space.

The Salvation Army requires the agility of a *movement* rather than the predictability of a machine. Working in more than 120 countries around the world, it faces varying configurations and pressures from the market and state demanding flexibility, agility, and alertness in the face of constantly changing circumstances.

ONE TELOS: "HEALTHY PERSONS"

The faithfulness of a *movement* can be sustained only through attention to matters of teleological orientation. Therefore, the second characteristic of Salvation Army health ministry is a *telos* of "healthy persons." Against the conception of people as "autonomous rational individuals," this book promotes an orientation towards "*healthy persons*" understood as "body-soul-in-relation." As noted earlier, the priority for "soul" over "body" in early Salvation Army practice resulted in some fragmentation of Salvation Army mission between corps and social—"body" work was left to the social services professionals and the corps focused on the work of saving and sanctifying souls. Such dualism was, and is, unfaithful and will require long-term attention for recovery.

There is evidence of Salvation Army practice and policy taking steps towards recovery. The Salvation Army's official doctrinal statements in recent years have emphasized the relational dimensions of the Trinity and of human personhood coupled with an explicit rejection of dualism.[4] This appreciation of the anthropology of persons as body-soul is helpful in resisting the commodification of people as merely "bodies" with no consideration to the importance of their eternal personhood. The integrated "body-soul" understanding of persons is also important in resisting the under-valuing of the body with a narrow evangelical priority to "go for souls."[5]

In the past decade, Salvation Army practice has been significantly enhanced by General John Gowans' three-legged definition of integrated

---

4. *The Salvation Army Handbook of Doctrine*, 243.

5. William Booth's quotation "Go for souls and go for the worst" is well known in Salvation Army circles and continues to be often quoted by Salvationists all around the world. It appeared in print for the first time in *The War Cry*, 16 November 1889.

mission. Gowans promoted the slogan "The Salvation Army exists to save souls, grow saints, and serve suffering humanity." In other words, faithful Salvation Army engagement in the world includes opportunities for people to enjoy salvation, sanctification, and service.

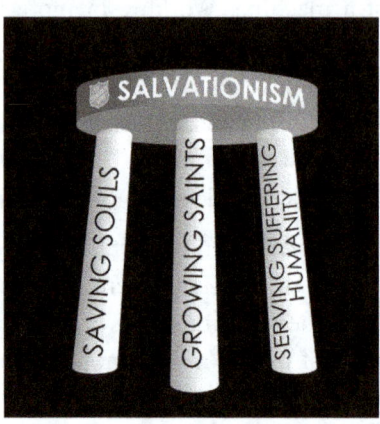

I have used Gowan's "three-legged stool" diagram in discussions around the world and find it helpful in challenging those who emphasize one "leg" while ignoring the other two—for example, the "sanctified" individualistic saint who has little time for "suffering humanity" or the passionate social worker who sees little need for connection between her professional practice and an eschatological *telos*.

General Linda Bond, the current international leader of The Salvation Army, built on the Gowans statement in setting out a vision for The Salvation Army after her election in 2011. Writing to her officers, Bond states: "We have *one mission*. Our mission is not three separate strands, assigned to certain sections of the Army. It is *one mission*. No part of the Army can divorce itself from serving suffering humanity. Nor can any part ignore the imperative to bring people to Jesus and make disciples."[6]

Gowans and Bond's understanding of Salvation Army mission is grounded in an anthropology of persons as body-soul and a Wesleyan teleological orientation towards perfection through the process of sanctification. Gowans and Bond resist any sectarian withdrawal by emphasizing the engagement in the world through the work of "serving suffering humanity." However, by keeping "serving suffering humanity" distinct, yet

---

6. Bond, "International Vision Statement," 4.

linked to salvation and sanctification, the ontological difference between the world and the Church is maintained while "service" is not reduced to simply a worthy end in itself.

A weakness in the Gowans statement is the lack of a relational dimension—his slogan can be read as focusing on the activity of individuals with no emphasis given to the importance of the relationships or working together. General Bond's slogan, "One Army, One Mission, One Message" has greater relational potential as it contains a strong emphasis on unity. Bond has been careful not to over define the way of achieving the vision—it has not been presented as a mechanistic prescription but rather calls people to move forward towards a vision of unity in organization, mission, and message. Bond defines the "message" in these words: "We need to effect change for people and can do so in many practical ways but only God in Jesus by his Spirit can make people new creatures in Christ, setting them free, giving them hope and life to the full."[7] As Rudman argued, life in all it fullness for a person must include both the rational and relational dimensions of personhood.[8] Bond's inclusion of a relational dimension, "One Army," could be a significant step in the recovery of Salvation Army practice from body-soul dualism but requires a more explicit articulation of the characteristics of people as "new creatures in Christ." Unsurprisingly, I hope such an articulation will be in accord with the *telos* of "healthy persons."

The strengthening of a relational focus in Salvation Army work has received significant attention from Salvation Army practitioners involved in "serving suffering humanity" in the past 30 years. The historical priority for practically "meeting needs" and "providing support" is still evident in many Salvation Army programs around the world. However, as noted in Needham's work in chapter 4, it is not enough to merely deliver services at social institutions such as hostels, hospitals or clinics. Relationship building is essential. Simply providing goods is an inadequate and unfaithful response if the potential for people as "body-soul-in-relation" is diminished in any way. Provision may meet body needs but can damage relationships and inhibit the soul-life. Power dynamics always need careful attention when "serving suffering humanity." The best people to respond to an issue are those affected by it—rather

---

7. Bond, "One Army, One Mission, One Message," 5.
8. Rudman, *Concepts of Person and Christian Ethics*, 171–89.

than those outside the situation wanting to help. Lessons learnt from a more relational way of working—particularly influenced by working with people affected by addictions, leprosy and HIV/AIDS—are further discussed later in this chapter.

HABITS AND PRACTICES

To sustain an orientation towards the *telos* of "healthy persons," the third characteristic required of a rightly orientated Salvation Army ministry requires theologically informed *habits and practices*. Such habits and practices are foundational to the work of people of faith wherever they are working albeit in hospitals, clinics, churches, or in households and communities. As noted in earlier field reflections, the dominant bio-medical models of health coupled with the commodification of health care pose significant risks to faith-based health ministry and, more importantly, the health of the poorest people. Medicine is not merely a work to "fix" the body or generate a profit. Rather, engaging with the quest for health and the fight against illness should be understood as opportunities to serve God's purposes in redeeming the fallen world.

Central to Hauerwas's response to illness and contemporary medicine has been a call for greater participation of human presence in the face of suffering. However, as Hauerwas argues, this participation needs to be sustained by the habits and practices of the church. During my visits to Salvation Army programs in the writing of this book, I noted practice—sustained by the habits and practices of faith—displaying the characteristics of "faithful presence" towards the *telos* of "healthy persons."

For example, in Bolivia, The Salvation Army hospital in Cochabamba is small with 48 beds in comparison to the hospitals in India and Indonesia, which have more than 200 beds. Like the Asian hospitals, the Cochabamba hospital does not receive state funding but depends on patient fees for the vast majority of its income. Despite pressure from commercial providers, The Salvation Army hospital covers its running costs by offering a quality, focused package of hospital-based care integrated with a community-based mobile clinic program. Financial profits made in the hospital help fund the community-based program. Clients mainly come from the poorer sections of Cochabamba society and The Salvation Army gives subsidies for people in extreme need. Subsidies can be given only after patients are reviewed by the chaplains who take time to discern the situation—rather than by clinical or administrative staff. There are a high number of practicing Christians on the staff—in addition to quality leadership from Salvation Army officers—and increasingly links are being strengthened with Salvation Army corps and other worshipping congregations in the area. The community health team visits the poorer areas of the city each day, often linking up with local churches, to offer a range of services including primary health care, income generation activities, and education programs for women and children.

The success of the program and the limitations of the existing building resulted in pressure to build a large multi-specialist facility. After much debate, the leaders decided to maintain the same number of in-patient beds but increase the capacity of the hospital to support community-based health work. Therefore, the number of outpatient consulting rooms more than doubled; the clinical support services (laboratory, x-ray, and pharmacy) improved and more space has been given to the community health team for offices and training facilities. A financial analysis before construction, and early results since completion, indicates that this model is financially sustainable. An analysis of the medical-health context shows the integrated health program offers an effective means to address the greatest health issues confronting the poorest people.

Throughout this time of change, attention was given to the importance of *process* in working through disagreements and potential conflicts by seeking to improve relationships between health staff, members of worshipping congregations and other partners such as the Bolivian State Health Department and universities. As a result, the various Salvation Army groups and other members of the community worked together to clarify the purpose of health ministry, developed a greater sense of shared mission, and strengthened systems complementing the new building project. This resulted in greater integration in habits and practice, which will sustain faithful orientation and faithful presence in the future.

Another example of faithful practice is in Ghana where The Salvation Army has a network of clinic-hospitals in rural and urban locations. Unlike Bolivia, India, and Indonesia, the government of Ghana provides significant funding. The funding of government and faith-based health services across Ghana has increased significantly in the past decade with the introduction of an ambitious state-led health insurance scheme funded by a Value Added Tax and employee social security contributions.[9] The scheme significantly improved levels of funding and, consequently, improved patient care in Salvation Army clinic-hospitals. However, this has brought increased pressure on Salvation Army leaders to expand the size of the clinic-hospitals into fully-fledged general hospitals. This pressure is being resisted but it is indicative of the dominance of the bio-medical framework that significant Ghanaian voices argue that progress can only be evidenced by larger hospitals and greater specialization.

Ghanaians pressing for the "development" of large hospitals appear not to appreciate the faithfulness of their existing health ministry. Probably the best example of faithful presence I have witnessed in any Salvation Army health program is the community-based program for children with disabilities supported by a small residential program at Begoro. A relatively small cluster of buildings in a rural setting provides physical rehabilitation for children plus support and training for the parents. Participating in a time of "praise and worship" with the children, parents, and staff was a deeply moving experience. I reflected later on the impact and importance that these simple habits and practices of faithfulness contribute to sustaining the day-to-day hard work that is health ministry.

The trained and experienced community rehabilitation staff regularly visits children with disabilities in their homes and help families and the people around them to deal with issues of discrimination and stigma. Community based support groups have been formed—often linked to local churches and mosques. Ghana has a substantial number of its citizens who are Muslim (approximately 15 percent of the population) and there is good cooperation at household and village level particularly on areas of mutual interest such as health. The Salvation Army programs are well used by Muslims and there is evidently a spirit of cooperation and collaboration between the faith-groups.

These two examples highlight the contribution of the *habits and practices* of people of faith upon health ministry in clinic-hospitals, congregations, communities, and households. Frameworks based on rational managerialism—underpinned by the notion of the "autonomous rational individual"—give little space for valuing the relational nature of persons. The effectiveness, efficiency, and "fixing" priorities tend to shut down

---

9. There is little published research on the impact of Ghana's health insurance scheme. An outline of the types of insurance is available at http://www.ghanaweb.com/GhanaHomePage/health/national_health_insurance_scheme.php.

the space. People of faith engaging in health ministry can create space by intentionally prioritizing practices—such as listening, conversations, hospitality, singing, praying—and, in so doing, discover capacity that the managerial frameworks under value. These are key aspects in the healing process towards being "healthy persons." In seeking such a *telos* supported by faithful practices, FBOs can be participants in the task of embedding medicine in social relations.

However, in my travels to many parts of the world, I regularly identify a lack of integration between a number of faith-based institutions—churches, schools, clinics, and hospitals—in a particular geographical location. Too often, Salvation Army social institutions appear to prioritize closer links with the respective government departments,[10] or regulatory bodies or focus on commercial priorities, rather than seeking a continuous chain of faith-based ministry focused on serving suffering humanity. To encourage discussion and imagining among practitioners, the following diagram was developed to illustrate the ideal of faith-based integrated health care based on shared *telos* and evidenced by deep relationships.

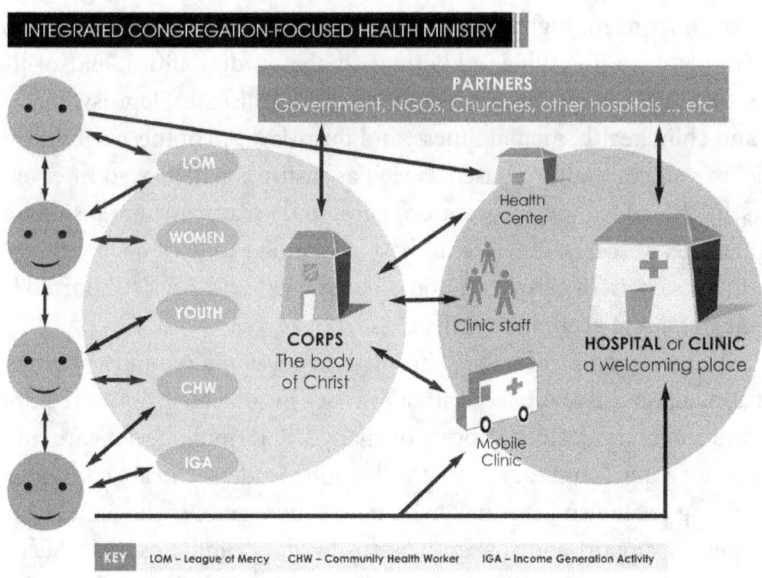

This model of integrated, socially embedded, health ministry gives primacy to responses as close to the family as possible supported

10. Ministry of Health or Education.

by quality relationships between the institutions of household, church, and hospital. The black arrow-lines are not incidental but are central in enabling all participants to develop a shared *telos*, which sustains often fragile relationships in chaotic communities. These are often fragile relationships requiring careful and ongoing attention.

As argued in Chapter 3, clinic-hospitals can be a significant support to congregation and community-based initiatives but they can also become distractions and diversions. Faith-based health ministry in the twenty-first century needs to shift its practice from prioritizing multi-specialist hospital services to a greater emphasis on primary health care as close to the family as possible. Implementing this shift will require prioritization of certain health interventions. It is not possible to meet every health need. Therefore, faith-based hospitals should focus on interventions to which they can best respond—according to capacity and context while retaining consideration on the orientation for "healthy persons."

In light of this, The Salvation Army has prioritized health practices with a "relational" dimension. In other words, medical conditions that benefit from long-term relationships as against those which generally require short-term, high technology interventions. The following list of conditions were identified: addictions, diabetes, disabilities, end-of-life care, eyes, HIV/AIDS, hypertension, infectious diseases, leprosy, maternal and child health, mental illness, and nutrition. All of these conditions benefit from community-based as well as institutionally based interventions in the education, prevention, care, and treatment dimensions of primary health care. They are all best responded to with an integrated, continuous chain of care from home-to-hospital-and-back supported by people of faith at every link of the chain.

The reorientation of mission hospitals in developing countries towards a relational, reflective process with a primary health care priority requires a significant and sustained process of change. Reforming health care ministry is not a quick and easy task. It will require leaders who are committed to building relationships with worshipping congregations who, in turn, are prepared to support and sustain tension-dwelling clinic-hospitals. Such a move opens up opportunities for congregation and clinic-hospitals to be "faithfully present" with families and individuals engaging in prevention, health promotion, home care, and rehabilitation initiatives as people take greater responsibility for their health. Central to the task is the work of building deeper relationships between "healthy persons."

There are risks in developing congregation-based health services. Firstly, the instrumentalization of health services is a particular risk for churches engaging in "direct health care" services. The "instrumental" attitude manifests itself in the congregations wanting to "do something" about the plight of "the poor" rather than commit to deep relationships with people. Thus, it is critically important that congregation-based health ministries (and other FBO health services) affirm, enhance, and appreciate the faith works of the poor themselves as they find both their agency and identity in the task of improving their own health. This emphasis embraces two important theological principles in developing further the account of "healthy persons" particularly for the poorest people who must be seen as both made in the image of God and called to be actors in the drama of creation and salvation itself.

A second area of concern is the trend by FBOs—encouraged by the funding priorities of government funders and secularist public health frameworks—to promote community-based health programs rather than congregation-based initiatives. FBOs developing health or development programs in a particular location may invite churches to participate but, often, only as one voice among many. There is little attention given to the importance of the habits and practices of faith or the clarity of their *telos*. Therefore, it is important that faith leaders are able to discern the *telos* of the funding agencies. Are funders promoting a secularizing concept of persons—such as the "autonomous rational individual" or are they creating space for the development of "healthy persons"? As argued earlier, a disagreement over *telos* does not preclude partnership but it should alert faith leaders to the dangers of institutional isomorphism.

In order to resist a drift towards any form of unfaithful *telos*, this book recommends every FBO and faith-based program is coupled with a worshipping congregation. This enables the habits and practices of the worshipping congregation to sustain the faithfulness of the service in, with and for "Babylon." Salvation Army worshipping congregations—often in corps but not exclusively—meet together regularly and are formed and sustained by the habits and practices such as reading the Bible, singing, testimonies, listening to music prayer and worship in the power of the Spirit. Hauerwas and Wells propose the liturgy as an ordered set of practices that shape the character and assumptions of the worshipping community of Christians. The liturgy, they suggest, offers habits and models that can inform every aspect of relational life such as "meeting people, acknowledging fault and failure, celebrating, thanking, reading, speaking with authority, reflecting on wisdom, naming truth, registering need, bringing about reconciliation, sharing food, and renewing purpose. This is the basic staple of Christian life—not simply for clergy or for those in religious orders, but for lay Christians, week in, week out."[11]

This reveals an interesting tension with Salvation Army theology and practice. By placing the traditional worship practices of Church at the center of his theology, Hauerwas emphasizes liturgy and sacrament as the unifying practices of Christ-followers. However, Salvationists do not observe the celebration of the Eucharist in worship, do not practice water baptism nor have a set liturgy. Hauerwas promotes the Eucharist as a powerful sign of the dependence of the church upon Christ. In contrast, Salvation Army theology and practice has emphasized dependence on the Holy Spirit. Hauerwas recently argued: "People do not drop from the sky but rather become who they are through training in practices that form the habits of hearts and tongues."[12] This quotation highlights the extent to which Hauerwas continues to undervalue the Spirit and the divine work of transformation that has been foundational in Salvation Army theology and ministry.

There is inadequate space here to discuss the doctrine and practice of "total sacramental living" in The Salvation Army. However, I witnessed Salvationist worship characterized by the same habits and practices promoted by Hauerwas, in addition to a reliance on the resources of the Spirit. Despite the rejection by the early Salvationists of the observance of formal, traditional forms of worship, Salvationists continued (and continue) to place importance on "meeting people, acknowledging fault and failure, celebrating, thanking, reading, speaking with authority, reflecting on wisdom, naming truth, registering need, bringing about reconciliation, sharing food, and renewing purpose." These are identifiable characteristics of Salvationist worship.[13] The Bible is central; preaching is valued; relationships with God and others are prioritized as purpose is renewed.

---

11. Hauerwas and Wells, "Christian Ethics as Informed Prayer," 7.

12. Hauerwas and Coles, *Christianity, Democracy and the Radical Ordinary*, 111.

13. Salvation Army worship developed traditions including a Holiness Meeting on Sunday morning and a Salvation Meeting on Sunday evening. This format is no longer as consistent as it was—however the practices Hauerwas promotes can be identified in almost all Salvation Army worship activities.

The first Salvationists believed it necessary to stop participating in the practices of liturgy and sacrament believing a reliance on "empty" rituals was unnecessary and prevented people experiencing fullness of life in the Holy Spirit. However, an over dependency on the work of the Spirit, it appears to me, has enabled a highly individualist conception of holiness to flourish in some Salvationists understanding of their faith. To a large extent, in the first century of The Salvation Army (1878 to 1978), this was mitigated by a strong sense of duty—part of being a Salvationist was a requirement to participate in the life of the corps. The concept of duty kept many Salvationists habitual. However, I note a changing understanding of what it means to be a committed Salvationist in the past 20 years—particularly in the western context. As duty has lost its power to sustain committed participation, an individualistic conception of holiness has allowed some to opt out of communal activities (including worship) as these seem unnecessary if the Holy Spirit can be as easily accessed on the golf course or via a podcast as at Sunday morning worship. This over confident pneumatology results in a loss of commitment to the community of believers due to a lack of appreciation for the habits and practices of worship.

Bretherton argues neither the worship habits nor social actions of the church and its members are adequate evidence to distinguish Christians from non-Christians. Rather the specific difference between the church and other communities is the nature of their different relationships with God: "Distinctiveness lies in how God is present to and within the church. Distinctiveness does not necessarily lie in what the church looks like or does . . . God is at work in all creation, and all may be justified in Christ; however, before the *parousia*, it is given particularly to the church to be the witness to, and the place of, transfigured social relations."[14] The significance of this statement for Salvation Army practice is that it highlights the importance not of ritual, habit, or duty but rather of relationships. A priority for relationships is a corrective to a highly individualistic holiness. It is not enough for a Christian to be right with God through the power of the Holy Spirit—there has to be evidence of "transfigured social relations." Equally, as the early Salvationists believed, it is not enough to participate in the ritual of the Eucharist—there has to be evidence of "transfigured social relations."

---

14. Bretherton, *Hospitality as Holiness*, 107–8.

Therefore, we can conclude that a faithfully present church and the lives of "healthy persons" within it are evidenced not by duty or ritual but by transformed social relations. As transformed social relations are sustained by the worshipping practices of Christian disciples, FBOs need to seek evidence of transformed social relations as an indicator of faithfulness in all forms of ministry—including health ministry.

PARTNERSHIPS FOR THE COMMON GOOD

The fourth characteristic of faithfully present Salvation Army health ministry is the building of partnerships based on "mutual interest" through a process of reflective practice. This book promotes a tradition-specific practical theological approach to health ministry. This goes against the dominant trend in interfaith dialogue where partnerships are sought around "shared values" such as "justice" and "human development." Indeed, some people perceive theology and the habits and practices of specific faith-groups to be potentially divisive.

Tony Blair, the former British Prime Minister, in a speech on faith and development, articulated a negative perception of tradition-specific theology in 2009. Blair argued: "When faith communities collaborate and work together for justice and human development there is a double pay off: things get done and respect and understanding between them grows. A dialogue that moves from hands to hearts to heads complements what is normally understood as inter-religious dialogue. A dialogue from heads to hearts does not always result in multi-faith action."[15]

Blair's concerns about the ineffectiveness of "inter-religious dialogue" are well founded. The best way to build a relationship across a faith-divide is not in the debating chamber. However, I am not convinced by his proposal to sideline the "head." It suggests an inadequate appreciation of the importance of the traditions, *telos*, habits, and practices that sustain all people of faith. As this book has argued, people of faith should not be left without a narrative to orientate their habits and practices. These are essential in the sustaining of a faithful presence. A lack of attention to *telos* will weaken FBOs and—in due course—limit their ability to contribute to improving the health of the poorest people leaving everyone vulnerable to the forces of institutional isomorphism.

---

15. Blair, "Launch Address."

The way forward, I propose, is the use of a process of reflective practice to enable people of different faiths to work and talk together by affirming and acknowledging the contribution of their faith without collapsing different theologies into a morass of commonality. Therefore, partnerships should be developed with the resources of practical theology to enhance and embed beliefs and practices rather than attempting to distance them. In response to Blair, I argue, it is necessary to bring "heads," "hands" and "hearts" to the cause of public health in an integrated process of mutual respect and common interest.

Having said that, Blair is right to promote the contribution of faith in practical tasks as it can be a particularly fruitful means of developing common ground between people of different teleological convictions. However, the expectation should not be that people leave their faith at home—but rather that a shared concern for the health of everyone in the community creates a space for engagement between people of different faiths. The following diagram has been helpful in stimulating discussion and legitimating inter-faith partnerships by Salvation Army health programs.

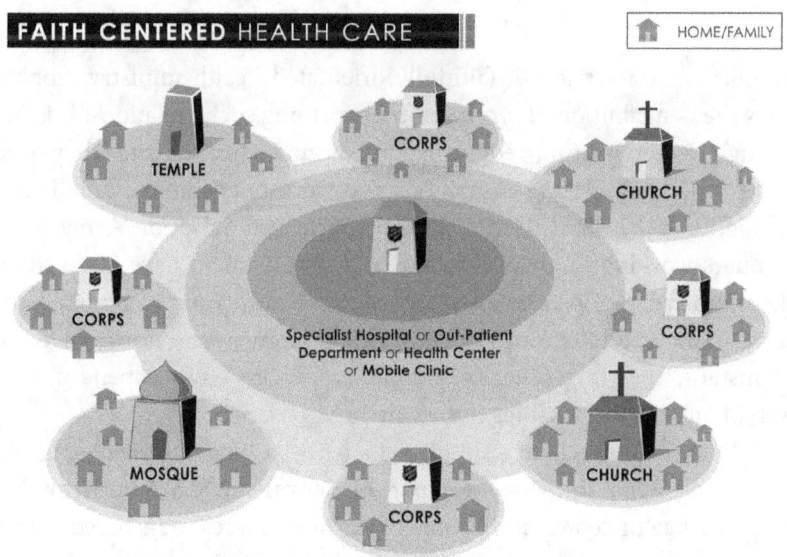

In this model, faith congregations maintain their distinctive traditions but come together at the health institution or health issue in a common response to a shared concern. Admittedly, this is an idealistic model and the reality is often an environment of contested and conflicting relations. However, experience has shown that barriers can be overcome and relationships developed if the process is properly facilitated. Hospitals and clinics offer space for dialogue and ultimately for relationship building as I witnessed in November 2011 in East Jerusalem at the Augusta Victoria Hospital on the Lutheran World Federation campus on the Mount of Olives. Christians, Muslims and Jews work together for the health of many poor and marginalized Palestinian people, despite many political, social, economic, and historical barriers. People of various faiths are not asked to leave their faith at home but rather to work together around an issue of mutual concern—the fight against cancer—characterized by hospitality, respect, and a determination to be faithful to their own particular traditions and teaching.

These relationships do not just happen, nor do they survive without careful attention. A process of relationship building is required to foster dialogue and bring congregation, community, and health professionals together. This brings us to the fifth characteristic of faithfully orientated health ministry.

FAITH-BASED PROCESS

The fifth characteristic of faithfully orientated health ministry emphasizes the contribution of *process* in transforming social relations. It is not enough to merely bring people together around a health issue. They need to be facilitated in their discussions and work to enable the building of strong, deep, resilient relationships. Experienced Salvation Army practitioners working in areas of health and development have understood the importance of *process* for many years. Health issues of mutual concern—such as addictions, HIV/AIDS, and leprosy—are not resolved in an instant. They take time. They require a process. They depend upon a web of quality relationships if they are to be beaten.

I observed excellent examples of a faith-based *process* way of working during a visit to the western part of Kenya. The Salvation Army has only one health center in this area but a vast congregation-based health ministry particularly supporting women and children infected and affected by HIV/AIDS. Almost all of the congregations function without support from health institutions and are able to engage in a significant health ministry by focusing on developing relationships through a structured process of home and community visits, listening activities, reflection, and discussion supported by a limited—but valued—input of health education and minimal treatment activities.

Groups work in rural and urban settings, based around congregations and include people of other faiths such as Muslims. The group decides what issues to focus on. For example, there are AIDS widows support groups, teenage health groups (focusing primarily on prevention messages), groups for mothers, babies, and toddlers as well as men's health groups. The groups use a common process way of working using basic facilitation skills, a regular self-assessment process and regular worship activities which helps retain a faith-distinctive character. Positive outcomes include improved health education, prevention of disease, and increased care and support activities as well as income generation activities to provide ongoing financial support for vulnerable group members. The women in these groups had not only learnt skills and gained knowledge, more importantly they gained confidence in their ability to grapple with their challenging circumstances. The women believe in themselves, each other and their way of working together in the group; they are determined to respond to their challenges and the small amounts of donor funding supporting some of their activities does not appear to be destabilizing the process to any significant extent.

In other field visits around the world, I have observed very different outcomes. Where donor funds and donor priorities are dominant factors in the process, there is almost always a lack—or loss—of ownership by the intended beneficiaries. Too often the approach of the external donors—working with a managerialist framework—reduces the capacity of people to respond to their situation. This is a problem for FBOs—including The Salvation Army—where there is a lack of consistency in the articulation of theologically informed practice particularly among "professional" employees. The "professional" *telos* is too often informed by secularist ideologies—influenced by an appreciation of autonomous, rational individuals—rather than by theologically informed ways of working. My review of the resources developed by The Salvation Army in the fields of community health and development in 2007 suggested too many frameworks for development were based on western secularist development models promoting "autonomous rational individuals" rather than an appreciation of "healthy persons." Therefore, the development of resources to enable a theologically informed way of understanding professional practice became a priority. How could the character and outcomes of the groups working in Kenya—and other places—be replicated across The Salvation Army?

Given the size and diversity of Salvation Army social work around the world, the resources have to be accessible to employees and volunteers who do not share the same theological perspectives but are willing to acknowledge that faith and spiritual experiences plays an important role in developing healthy people. Theological reflection models offered a connection point with cyclical process models used in many areas of professional practice such as the learning cycle, the planning cycle, and the care management cycle. Therefore, a process way of working which validated faith-commitment and theological ways of thinking based on the pastoral cycle was developed.

I identified another connection point between FBO and secular development practice in the use of facilitation methods and tools. The practice of facilitation in The Salvation Army has been widely advocated for a number of years, but it was unclear the degree to which this practice had been theologically grounded. Facilitation is an approach widely used by secular agencies as well as FBOs. In its secularist guise, it claims to enable people to think for themselves and develop solutions from their own resources. Some Salvation Army practitioners justify the use of facilitation on this basis and appeared to be promoting an overconfident faith in the individual's capacity to solve their problems.

However, on field visits such as the time in Kenya, I observed many practitioners using facilitation tools but infusing them with faith-based insights and perspectives. In this application, facilitation displayed many of the characteristics of faithful presence such as hospitality and listening. This way of working opened up space for transfigured social relations when it meaningfully engaged with church practices such as Bible reading, prayer, and reflection. I noted facilitation being used as a means of building healthy relationships with people within and outside of the church. However, while some faith-based facilitators were skilled in their practice, they were rarely able to articulate this way of working or successfully replicate it across the organization. This relationally dependent way of working was very effective in a few places but was inevitably undermined by a change of personnel or other disrupting factors.

During 2009, at my request, The Salvation Army engaged The Oxford Centre for Ecclesiology and Practical Theology (OXCEPT) to assist in the development of a resource for field workers. Judith Thompson, author of a book on Theological Reflection[16] took the lead in writing the text using practical examples some of which came from my field reflection notes. Her model of theological reflection—based on the Pastoral Cycle—was adapted by a group of experienced Salvation Army practitioners to increase its resonance and relevance with field-based practitioners. The term Faith-Based Facilitation was coined to describe the adapted process.

The team of Salvation Army practitioners worked with OXCEPT colleagues and developed the following definition and diagram to explain the process and purpose of Faith-Based Facilitation: "Faith-Based Facilitation a process and a set of tools which helps, encourages, and enables people to speak and, in the light of Biblical truths, make more faithful decisions and enjoy deeper relationships. An intentional searching for spiritual insight (called "*Kairos* Experience") is central to Faith-Based Facilitation. A facilitator does not only have skills and tools, s/he seeks a Christ-like character."

The Faith-Based Facilitation (FBF) process includes the four key elements of the Wesleyan Quadrilateral—Scripture, Tradition, Reason, and Experience—but by adopting the action-reflection process it is more recognizable to people familiar with secular models. While the five-stage process is widely used, the recognition of the influence of Bible, Faith Tradition, and the work of the Spirit (*Kairos* Experience) makes it distinctively faith-based.

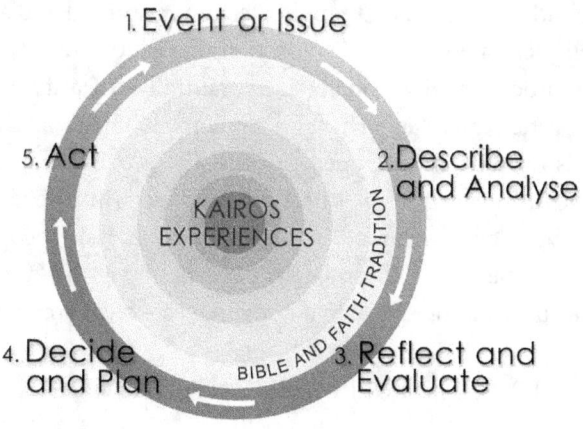

16. Thompson, *SCM Studyguide for Theological Reflection*.

The FBF process starts when people identify something that requires attention (*Stage 1: Issue or Event*). It might be a significant concern, or a regular pattern of activity that needs to be carefully examined to see "what we are doing and why we are doing it." Whatever it is, the experience needs to be clearly identified—preferably by a group of people working together—to agree the issue or event. The experience and lessons learnt by Salvation Army facilitators in the past 15 years are particularly important at this stage and Stage 2. The power dynamics must be carefully analyzed. If the issues are being identified or imposed from outside of the group, the change is unlikely to be sustainable or faithful.

The experience of the people affected by the issue is then described and analyzed as fully as possible in Stage 2 (*Describe and Analyze*). Those who are reflecting (together or individually) are encouraged to identify every factor that is impacting the issue being explored. This contributes to the development of as comprehensive a description as possible of the issue or event under consideration. Facilitators are encouraged to remain as objective as possible by paying careful attention to description and analysis while avoiding judgments and opinions. A range of tools can be used at this stage as the group explores the issue or event as fully as possible.

The third stage of the process involves thinking through the factors that have emerged, sharing ideas, and responses (*Reflect and Evaluate*). The importance of Scriptures, prayer, and quiet reflection as helpful activities for people of faith is emphasized. Tools assisting a process of careful evaluation are used and tough questions are asked and answered.

A well-facilitated time of reflection based on the Faith-Based Facilitation process will normally lead naturally towards a decision, which the participants can own, and implement (Stage 4: *Decide and Plan*). Tools have been developed to assist the process if agreement is difficult. The fifth stage translates decisions and plans into deeds (*Action*). Again tools have been included in the resource to assist people at this stage. Like all cycles, the FBF process, does not stop at the last stage, but continues around another cycle in an ongoing reflective process.

TOOLS TO SUPPORT THE FBF PROCESS

The FBF process is supported by a wide range of tools to assist participants develop a comprehensive understanding and response. Simple tools such as listening, exploring, community walks, and visits, community mapping, brainstorming, prioritizing, creative thinking, problem solving, and self-assessment tools are highly effective in the hands of a skilled faith-based facilitator. These are only a few examples from the wide range of helpful tools. Other tools from the social and natural sciences can be used to give particular insights depending on the issue or event under review.

The FBF process and tools are now being used around the world in a range of situations, which benefit from a reflective process. These include an adult education session particularly around behavior change (learning); a home or community visit (caring); a problem-solving session with a group or an individual (counseling); helping a group or organization write a plan (planning); and developing a "Christian voice" to engage with wider society (advocacy). A common outcome is the building of deeper relationships.

A booklet explaining the FBF process and tools, *Building Deeper Relationships*, has been translated into a number of languages including French, Spanish, Swahili, Mandarin, Indonesian, Hindi, and Chichewa.[17] The title captures the priority for the work of all FBOs—their greatest contribution is not through technical tools or biomedical interventions. The most important work for FBOs is the building of deeper relationships.

CONCLUSION

In closing, I propose three areas for further work. Firstly, this is a modest attempt at a piece of global practical theology. However, it has highlighted the importance and value of attempting practical theology with a global perspective and the dangers of practice (and theology) being culturally limited. The global context of the twenty-first century will require leaders of all faiths to pay greater attention to global practical theology. Each tradition needs clarity on their *telos* and the framework, processes, habits, and practices that sustain that *telos*. Out of this comes opportunities and confidence to build partnerships with people with alternative priorities. Every tradition needs to use a reflective process to enable partnership without assimilation. Such a tradition-specific approach to development needs to be accepted and encouraged particularly

---

17. For more information on *Building Deeper Relationships using Faith-Based Facilitation* visit www.salvationarmy.org/fbf. Copies of the booklet in a number of languages are available for download.

by the large donor agencies whose current ways of working—imposing western managerial frameworks for development—lack an appreciation of faith and cultural difference. In contrast, a faith-based facilitation way of working—using the resources of practical theology—offers an inclusive, yet tradition specific, approach resulting in the building of deeper, more resilient relationships.

Secondly, greater evidence is required to show that FBO's produce quality health outcomes. This book makes a theological argument informed by field reflections but greater documentation and evidence is required to develop a convincing body of evidence to endorse the *telos* of "healthy persons" over and against the current priority for "autonomous rational individuals." At present, the market-state, dominant in much of the world, will partner if FBOs justify their contribution on instrumental grounds. FBOs will probably need to accept these terms and partner for the common good. However, the challenge for FBOs will be providing instrumental evidence without becoming mere instruments of the market-state.

Thirdly, there is significant research at present by social scientists into the impact of FBOs but most of it fails to engage with theological resources. The premise of this book is that people of faith are more effective, efficient, and resilient when the resources of faith are explicitly acknowledged and relied upon. The resources of practical theology—working across the disciplines of theology and the social sciences—can assist people of faith to respond faithfully to the task of improving the health of the poorest people on Earth.

In light of this reflection on practice, I conclude that Salvation Army health ministry in the twenty-first century—and other FBOs—should seek the characteristics of *movement* for the development of *"healthy persons,"* who are formed and sustained by the *habits and practices* of worshipping congregations in the power of the Spirit, who support clinic-hospitals, households, and other institutions and groups with a *theologically reflective* process way of working, resulting in faithful presence, and the transformation of *social relations* as God intends.

Bibliography and References

African Conference of Health Ministers. *African Health Strategy (2007 to 2015)—Strengthening Health Systems for Equity and Development in Africa*. Johannesburg: African Union, 2007.
Akin, John. *Financing Health Services in Developing Countries*. Washington DC: The World Bank, 1987.
Atherton, John, et al. *Christianity and the New Social Order—A manifesto for a fairer future*. London: SPCK, 2011.
Augustine. *The City Of God Against The Pagans*. Cambridge: Cambridge University Press, 1998.
AUSAID. *Helping Health Systems Deliver—A Policy for Australian Development Assistance in Health*. Canberra: The Australian Agency for International Development, 2006.
Baker, Christopher, and John Reader. *Entering The New Theological Space: Blurred Encounters of Faith, Politics and Community*. Farnham: Ashgate, 2009.
Bane, Mary Jo, el al. *Taking Faith Seriously*. Cambridge, MA: Harvard University Press, 2005.
Bano, Masooda and Padmaja Nair. "Faith Based Organizations in South Asia: Historical Evolution, Current Status and Nature of Interaction with the State." *Religion and Development Research Programme Working Paper 12*, International Development Department, University of Birmingham (2007).
Barnighausen, Till and Rainer Sauerborn. "One Hundred And Eighteen Years of the German Health Insurance System: Are There Any Lessons For Middle- and Low-income Countries?" *Social Science and Medicine* 54, 10 (2002) 1559–87.
Bebbington, D. W. "Atonement, Sun and Empire 1880 to 1914," in *The Imperial Horizons of British Protestant Missions 1880 to 1914*, edited by Andrew Porter. Grand Rapids, Michigan: Wm. B. Eermans Publishing Co, 2003.
Begbie, Harold. *Life of William Booth—The Founder of The Salvation Army* (Volume Two). London: MacMillan and Co, 1920.
Benedict. *The Rule of St. Benedict*. New York: Vintage Books, 1998.
Benton, Kerry William. "Saints and Sinners: Training Papua New Guinean (PNG) Christian Clergy to Respond to HIV and AIDS Using a Model of Care." *Journal of Religion and Health* 47, (2008) 314–25.
Bevans, Stephen. *An Introduction to Theology in Global Perspectives*. Maryknoll, NY: Orbis Books, 2009.

Biggar, Nigel. "Is Stanley Hauerwas Sectarian?" In *Faithfulness and Fortitude: Conversations with the Theological Ethics of Stanley Hauerwas,* edited by Mark Nation et al., 141–60. Edinburgh: T. & T. Clark, 2000.

Birungi, H. "Injections and Self-Help: Risk and Trust in Ugandan Health Care." *Social Science and Medicine,* 47, 10 (1998) 1455–62.

Blair, Tony. "Launch Address." Paper presented at Faith and Development Seminar Series. The Royal Society for the Encouragement of Arts, Manufacturers and Commerce, London, September 7, 2009.

Blas, Erik and M. E. Limbambala. "The Challenge of Hospitals in Health Sector Reform: The Case of Zambia." *Health Policy Plan.* 16, 2 (2001) 29–43.

Block, Fred. "Introduction to The Great Transformation," in *The Great Transformation—The Political and Economic Origins of our Time* by Karl Polanyi. xviii–xxxviii. Boston, MA: Beacon Press, 2001.

Bolger, Joe, el al. *Papua New Guinea's Health Sector: A Review of Capacity, Change and Performance Issues.* Maastricht: The Netherlands, European Centre for Development Policy Management, 2005.

Bond, Linda. "International Vision Statement," *The Officer,* July–August (2011) 4–5.

Bond, Linda. "One Army, One Mission, One Message," *The Officer,* September–October (2011) 4–5.

Booth-Tucker, Frederick. *The Life of Catherine Booth—The Mother of The Salvation Army.* London: The Salvation Army, 1892.

Booth, Bramwell. Personal Communication with William Booth. London: Salvation Army Heritage Centre, 1907.

———. "The General's Address" in *The International Social Council, 1921.* 1–55. London: The Salvation Army, International Headquarters, 1921.

Booth, Catherine. "Filled With The Spirit" in *Papers on Aggressive Christianity* Address 8, 1–14 London: The Salvation Army, 1880.

———. *Godliness: Addresses on Holiness, Exeter Hall.* London: The Salvation Army, 1881.

Booth, William. "Salvation For Both Worlds," *All The World* V, 1 (1889) 1 6.

———. *In Darkest England And The Way Out.* London: The Salvation Army, 1890.

———. "The Millenium—The Ultimate Triumph of Salvation Army Principles," *All The World* VI, 8 (1890) 337–43.

———. *A Letter from The General—To The Officers of The Salvation Army Throughout the World on the Occasion of his Eightieth Birthday.* London: The Salvation Army, 1909.

———. The Principles of Social Work (Part 1). In *International Social Council, 1911.* 14–31. St Albans: The Salvation Army, 1911.

Bossert, Thomas J., and Joel C. Beauvais. "Decentralization of Health Systems in Ghana, Zambia, Uganda and the Philippines: A Comparative Analysis of Decision Space." *Health Policy Plan.* 17, 1 (2002) 14–31.

Bretherton, Luke. *Hospitality as Holiness: Christian Witness amid Moral Diversity.* Aldershot: Ashgate, 2006.

———. "A Postsecular Politics? Inter Faith Relations as a Civic Practice." Paper presented at The Lambeth Inter Faith Lecture, Lambeth Palace, June 4, 2009.

———. *Christianity and Contemporary Politics.* Chichester: Wiley-Blackwell, 2010.

Brock, Brian. *Christian Ethics In A Technological Age.* Grand Rapids, Michigan: Wm. B. Eerdmans, 2010.

Calvert, Graham. *Health, Healing and Wholeness.* London: The Salvation Army, 1997.

Caspary, Almut. "On Health—A Critical Comparison of Contemporary Philosophical and Early Christian Interpretations of the Concept of Health in the Context of UK Human Embryonic Stem Cell Research Policies." PhD diss., King's College London, 2007.

Cavanaugh, William. *Theopolitical Imagination: Discovering the Liturgy as a Political Act in an Age of Global Consumerism.* London: T. & T. Clark, 2002.

Center for Global Development. *Does The IMF Constrain Health Spending In Poor Countries? Evidence and An Agenda for Action.* Washington DC: Center for Global Development, 2007.

Chand, Sarla and Jacqui Pattison. *Faith Based Models for Improving Maternal and New Born Health.* Washington DC: Access Programme for USAID, 2007.

Chansa, Collins, et al. "Exploring SWAp's Contribution to the Efficient Allocation and Use of Resources in the Health Sector in Zambia." *Health Policy Plan.* 23, 4 (2008) 244–51.

Clarke, Gerard. "Faith Matters: Development and the Complex World of Faith-Based Organizations." Paper presented at the annual conference of the Development Studies Association, Milton Keynes, September 7–9, 2005.

Collier, Paul. *The Bottom Billion: Why the poorest countries are failing and what can be done about it?* Oxford: Oxford University Press, 2007.

Coutts, John. *The Salvationists.* Oxford: Mowbrays, 1977.

Crespo, Richard. *The Future of Christian Hospitals in Developing Countries: The Call for a New Paradigm of Ministry.* Washington DC: Christian Connections for International Health, 2001.

Crisp, Nigel. "Global Health Partnerships: The UK Contribution to Health in Developing Countries." *Public Policy and Administration* 23, 2 (2008) 207–13.

Dale, Gareth. *Karl Polanyi—The Limits of the Market.* Cambridge, UK: Polity Press, 2010.

Das, Jishnu and Jeffrey Hammer. "Money For Nothing: The Dire Straits Of Medical Practice in Delhi, India." *Journal of Development Economics* 83, 1 (2007) 1–36.

Davies, H. "Falling Public Trust In Health Services: Implications For Accountability." *Journal of Health Services Research and Policy* 4 (1999) 193–94.

de Gruchy, Steve. "Of Agency, Assets and Appreciation: Seeking Some Commonalities Between Theology and Development." *Journal of Theology for Southern Africa* 117 (2003) 20–39.

de Kadt, Emanuel. "On Keeping God Out of Development." Paper presented at Development Studies Association Conference, 2008 "Development's Invisible Hands," Church House, Westminster, London, November 8, 2008.

Denscombe, Martyn. *The Good Research Guide: For Small-Scale Social Research Projects.* Maidenhead: Open University Press, 2003.

DFID. *Religion 'Good for Development'.* Department for International Development, Last Updated Date 2009 [cited 19 February 2010]. Available from http://www.developments.org.uk/articles/religion-2018good-for-development.

Di Maggio PJ and WW Powell. "The Iron Cage Revisited: Institutional Isomorphism and Collective Rationality in Organizational Fields." *American Sociological Review* 48, 2 (1983) 147–60.

Dibble, Susan. "The Salvation Army—The Search of a Wholistic Ministry. A Study of the Relationship Between its Evangelism and Social Service." MTh Diss., Northern Baptist Theological Seminary, 1991.

Easterly, William. *The White Man's Burden—Why the West's Efforts to Aid the Rest Have Done So Much Ill and So Little Good*. New York: Penguin, 2006.

Ekman, Bjorn. "Catastrophic Health Payments and Health Insurance: Some Counterintuitive Evidence from One Low-Income Country." *Health Policy* 83, 2–3 (2007) 304–13.

Ensor, Tim and Jeptepkeny Ronoh. "Effective Financing Of Maternal Health Services: A Review of the Literature." *Health Policy* 75, (2005) 49–58.

Etzioni, Amitai. "Communitarianism." In *From the Village to the Virtual World*, edited by Karen Christensen et al., 224–28. London: Sage Publications, 2003.

Evans, Abigail Rian. *The Healing Church—Practical Programs for Health Ministries*. Cleveland, Ohio: United Church Press, 1999.

Evers, Adalbert. "Part of the Welfare Mix: The Third Sector as an Intermediate Area." *Voluntas* 6, 2 (1995) 159–82.

Evers, Adalbert, and Jean-Louis Laville. *The Third Sector in Europe*. Cheltenham: Edward Elgar Publishing Limited, 2004.

Faguet, Jean-Paul, and Zulfiqar Ali. "Making Reform Work: Institutions, Dispositions, and the Improving Health of Bangladesh." *World Development* 37, 1 (2009) 208–18.

Felleman, Laura B. "A Necessary Relationship—John Wesley and the Body-Soul Connection." In *Inward and Outward Health: John Wesley's Holistic Concept of Medical Science, the Environment and Holy Living*, edited by Deborah Madden, 140–68. London: Epworth, 2008.

Fergusson, David. *Community, Liberalism and Christian Ethics*. New Studies in Christian Ethics. Cambridge: Cambridge University Press, 1998.

Flaws, Bonnie. "The Church in Papua New Guinea: A Blessing or a Curse? The Pros and Cons of Religion in Development." *Just Change* 6 (2006) 3–4.

Garlick, Phyllis. *The Wholeness of Man: A Study in the History of Healing*. London: Highway Press, 1943.

Gifford, Paul. *Christianity, Politics and Public Life in Kenya*. London: Hurst, 2009.

Gilson, Lucy. "Trust and the Development of Health Care as a Social Institution." *Social Science and Medicine* 56, 7 (2003) 1453–68.

Glenn, Charles L. *The Ambiguous Embrace: Government and Faith-Based Schools and Social Agencies*. Princeton, NJ: Princeton University Press, 2000.

Graham, Elaine, et al. *Theological Reflection: Methods*. London: SCM Press, 2005.

Green, Roger. *The Life and Ministry of William Booth*. Nashville, TN: Abingdon Press, 2005.

Grundmann, Christoffer H. *Sent To Heal! Emergence and Development of Medical Missions*. Lanham, Maryland: University Press of America, 2005.

Gunton, Colin. "Trinity, Ontology and Anthropology: Towards a Renewal of the Doctrine of the *Imago Dei*," in *Persons, Divine and Human—King's College Essays in Theological Anthropology*, edited by Christoph Schwobel et al. Edinburgh: T. & T. Clark, 1991.

Haddad, Barbara, et al. *The Potential and Perils of Partnership*. London: Tearfund, 2008.

Hall, John and Richard Taylor. "Health For All Beyond 2000: The Demise of the Alma-Ata Declaration and Primary Health Care in Developing Countries." *Medical Journal of Australia* 178 (2003) 17–20.

Hanson, Kara, et al. "Towards Improving Hospital Performance in Uganda and Zambia: Reflections And Opportunities For Autonomy." *Health Policy* 61, 1 (2002) 73–94.

Hattersley, Roy. *Blood And Fire: The Story of William and Catherine Booth and their Salvation Army*. London: Little, Brown, 1999.

Hauck, Volker, et al. *Ringing The Church Bell—The Role of Churches in Governance and Public Performance in Papua New-Guinea*. Maastricht, The Netherlands: European Centre for Development Policy Management, 2005.

Hauerwas, Stanley. *A Community Of Character: Toward A Constructive Christian Social Ethic*. London: University of Notre Dame Press, 1981.

———. "The Servant Community—Christian Social Ethics (1983)." In *The Hauerwas Reader*, edited by John Berkman et al., 371–91. Durham: Duke University Press, 2001.

———. "Why Medicine Needs the Church (1985)." In *The Hauerwas Reader*, edited by John Berkman et al., 539–55. Durham: Duke University Press, 2001.

———. *After Christendom?: How the Church is to Behave if Freedom, Justice, and a Christian Nation are Bad Ideas*. Nashville: Abingdon Press, 1991.

———. *Sanctify Them In The Truth: Holiness Exemplified*. Edinburgh: T. & T. Clark, 1998.

———. "How Christians Should Be Sick (1997)." In *The Hauerwas Reader*, edited by John Berkman et al., 348–66. Durham: Duke University Press, 2001.

———. "A Retrospective Assessment of an 'Ethics of Character': The Development of Hauerwas's Theological Project (1985, 2001)." In *The Hauerwas Reader*, edited by John Berkman et al., 75–89. Durham: Duke University Press, 2001.

Hauerwas, Stanley and Romand Coles. *Christianity, Democracy and the Radical Ordinary—Conversations between a Radical Democrat and a Christian*. Eugene, OR: Cascade Books, 2008.

Hauerwas, Stanley and Samuel Wells. "Christian Ethics as Informed Prayer." In *The Blackwell Companion to Christian Ethics*, edited by Stanley Hauerwas et al., 3–12. Oxford: Blackwell Publishing, 2004.

Higgins, Edward. "Unity of Operations in 'Aspects of Social Work in The Salvation Army.'" In *International Social Council, 1911*, 1–9. London: The Salvation Army, 1911.

Himmelfarb, Gertrude. *Poverty and Compassion: The Moral Imagination of the Late Victorians*. New York: Vintage Books, Random House, 1992.

Holmes, Stephen. "Introduction." In *Public Theology in Cultural Engagement*, edited by Stephen Holmes, 3–12. Milton Keynes: Paternoster, 2008.

Holmwood, John. "Three Pillars of Welfare State Theory: T.H. Marshall et al in Defence of the National Welfare State." *European Journal of Social Theory* 3, 1 (2000) 23–50.

Hovey, Craig. "Putting Truth To Practice: Macintyre's Unexpected Rule." *Studies in Christian Ethics* 19, 2 (2006) 169–86.

Howard, T Henry. "Spiritual Standards." In *International Social Council, 1911*. 217–27. London: The Salvation Army, 1911.

Howe, Brian. "Politics and Faith: Living in Truth." In *Church and Civil Society: A Theology of Engagement*, edited by Sue Leppert et al., Adelaide: ATF Press, 2004.

Hunter, James Davison. *To Change The World—The Irony, Tragedy and Possibility of Christianity in The Late Modern World*. New York: Oxford University Press, 2010.

Isaksen, Lise Widding, et al. "Global Care Crisis: A Problem of Capital, Care Chain, or Commons?" *American Behavioral Scientist* 52, 3 (2008) 405–25.

Islam, Anwar, and Tahir M. Zaffar. "Health Sector Reform in South Asia: New Challenges and Constraints." *Health Policy* 60, 2 (2002) 151–69.

Janisch, C. P., et al. "Demand Side Financing for Health Services." Paper presented at 35th Annual Global Conference for International Health. Washington DC, May 2008.

Jaya Shroff Bhalla. "Hospitals 'Blatantly' Flout Supreme Court Ruling." *Hindustan Times* 2010.

Jeavons, Thomas. *When The Bottom Line is Faithfulness: Management of Christian Service Organizations*. Bloomington: Indiana University Press, 1994.

Keating, P. J. *Into Unknown England, 1866–1913: Selections from the Social Explorers*. London: Fontana, 1976.

Kennedy, Sheila Suess. "Privatization And Prayer: The Challenge of Charitable Choice." *The American Review of Public Administration* 33, 1 (2003) 5-19.

Lawson, Kenneth. "William Booth's Darkest England Scheme: Christian Social Action Or Religious Opportunism?." BA diss., Leeds Metropolitan University, 1993.

MacIntyre, Alasdair C. *Whose Justice? Which Rationality?* Notre Dame, IN: University of Notre Dame Press, 1988.

———. *After Virtue: A Study In Moral Theory*. London: Gerald Duckworth and Co, 2007.

Macwan'gi, Mubiana and Alasford Ngwengwe. *Effectiveness of District Health Boards in Interceding for The Community*. Lusaka, The Institute of Economic and Social Research, The University of Zambia, 2004

Maddox, Randy L. *Responsible Grace: John Wesley's Practical Theology*. Nashville, Tenn.: Kingswood Books, 1994.

McArdle, Patrick. "The Relational Person Within a Practical Theology Of Health Care." PhD diss., Australian Catholic University, 2006.

McNiff, Jean, et al. *You And Your Action Research Project*. London: RoutledgeFalmer, 2003.

Mehrotra, Santosh and Enrique Delamonica. "The Private Sector and Privatization in Social Services: Is the Washington Consensus 'Dead'?" *Global Social Policy* 5, 2 (2005) 141–74.

Monsma, Stephen V. and Christopher Soper. *The Challenge of Pluralism: Church and State in Five Democracies*. Oxford: Rowman and Littlefield, 1997.

Montiel, Hector Cuadra. "Incompleteness of Post-Washington Consensus: A Critique of Macro-economic and Institutional Reforms." *International Studies* 44, 2 (2007) 103–22.

Murdoch, Norman H. *Origins of the Salvation Army*. Knoxville: University of Tennessee Press, 1994.

Nagel, Alexander-Kenneth. "Charitable Choices: The Religious Component on the US Welfare Reform—Theoretical and Methodological Reflections on Faith-Based Organizations as Social Service Agencies." *Numen* 53 (2006) 78–111.

Narvaez, Darcia and Daniel K. Lapsley. *Personality, Identity, and Character: Explorations in Moral Psychology*. New York: Cambridge University Press, 2009.

Needham, Philip. "Towards A Re-Integration of the Salvationist Mission." In *Creed and Deed—Towards a Christian Theology of Social Services in The Salvation Army*, edited by John D Waldron, 123–60. Oakville, Ontario: The Salvation Army Canada and Bermuda, 1986.

———. *Community In Mission—A Salvationist Ecclesiology*. London: The Salvation Army, 1987.

———. "The Theology: The Healing Gospel, The Healing Mission, The Healing Congregation," In *Health, Healing and Wholeness—Salvationist Perspectives*, edited by Graham Calvert. 25–66. London: The Salvation Army, 1997.

———. "Integrating Holiness and Community: The Task of an Evolving Salvation Army." *Word and Deed—A Journal of Salvation Army Theology and Ministry*. (2000).

Olivier, Jill. "In Search of Common Ground for Interdisciplinary Collaboration and Communication: Mapping the Cultural Politics of Religion and HIV/AIDS in Sub Saharan Africa." PhD diss., University of Cape Town, 2010.

Olivier, Jill, et al. *Working In A Bounded Field Of Unknowing—African Religious Health Assets Programme Literature Review*. Cape Town: University of Cape Town, 2006.
Omar, Khalid, "Hinduising India: Secularism in Practice." *Third World Quarterly* 29, 8, (2008) 1545–62.
Ott, Philip W. "John Wesley on Health as Wholeness." *Journal of Religion and Health* 30, 1 (1991) 43–57.
Pattison, Stephen and James Woodward. "Introduction to Pastoral and Practical Theology" in *The Blackwell Reader In Pastoral And Practical Theology*, edited by James Woodward et al., 1–19. Oxford: Blackwell Publishers, 2000.
Plant, Stephen, J. "Freedom as Development: Christian Mission and The Definition of Human Well-Being." Paper presented at Henry Martyn Seminar, Westminster College, Cambridge, 2002.
———. "Does Faith Matter In Development?" Paper presented at Faith and Development: Theory and Practice Forum, Cambridge, November 26–27, 2004.
———. "International Development and Belief in Progress." *Journal of International Development* 21, 6 (2009) 844–55.
Polanyi, Karl. *The Great Transformation—The Political and Economic Origins of our Time*. Boston, MA: Beacon Press, 2001.
Putnam, Robert D. *Bowling Alone. The Collapse And Revival of American Community*. New York: Simon & Schuster, 2000.
Railton, George Scott. *The Salvation Army Following Christ*. Atlanta (1986): The Salvation Army, 1907.
Reich, Michael R. "Reshaping The State From Above, From Within, From Below: Implications for Public Health." *Social Science and Medicine* 54 (2002) 1669–75.
Reinikka, Rivita and Jakob Svensson. *Working for God? Evaluating Service Delivery of Religious Not-for-Profit Health Care Providers in Uganda*. Washington DC, World Bank Publications, 2003.
Reno, R. R. "Stanley Hauerwas," in *The Blackwell Companion to Political Theology*, edited by Peter Scott et al., 302–16. Oxford: Blackwell Publishing, 2004.
Robinson, Barbara. "Bodily Compassion: Values and Identity Formation in The Salvation Army, 1880 to 1900." PhD Diss., The University of Ottawa, 1999.
Rudman, Stanley. *Concepts of Person and Christian Ethics*. New Studies in Christian Ethics. Cambridge: Cambridge University Press, 1997.
Sachs, Jeffrey. "Health In The Developing World—Achieving the Millennium Development Goals." *Bulletin of the World Health Organization* 82 (2004) 947–52.
Saith, A. "From Universal Values to MDGs: Lost in Translation." *Development and Change* 37, 6 (2007) 1167–99.
Sandall, Robert. *The History of The Salvation Army, Volume Three—Social Reform and Welfare Work*. Edinburgh: Thomas Nelson and Son, 1955.
Schiber, George, et al. "Financing Global Health: Mission Unaccomplished." *Health Affairs* 26, 4 (2007).
Schön, Donald A. *The Reflective Practitioner: How Professionals Think In Action*. Aldershot: Avebury, 1991.
Schwab, Linda S. "This Curious and Important Subject," in *Inward and Outward Health: John Wesley's Holistic Concept of Medical Science, the Environment and Holy Living*, edited by Deborah Madden, 169–212. London: Epworth, 2008.

Schwöbel, Christoph. "Introduction," in *Persons, Divine and Human—King's College Essays in Theological Anthropology*, edited by Christoph Schwobel et al. Edinburgh: T. & T. Clark, 1991.

Segall, M. "From Cooperation to Competition in National Health Systems—and Back? Impact on Professional Ethics and Quality of Care." *International Journal of Health Planning and Management* 15 (2000) 61–79.

Shaikh, B, et al. "Health Care and Public Health in South Asia." *Public Health* 120, 2 (2006) 142–44.

Shiffman, Jeremy. "Has Donor Prioritization of HIV/AIDS Displaced Aid for Other Health Issues?" *Health Policy Plan* 23, 2 (2008) 95–100.

Sider, Ronald J. and Heidi Rolland Unruh. "Typology of Religious Characteristics of Social Service and Educational Organizations and Programs." *Nonprofit and Voluntary Sector Quarterly* 33, 1 (2004) 109–34.

Silver, Beverly J and Giovanni Arrighi. "Polanyi's "Double Movement": The Belle Époques of British and U.S. Hegemony Compared." *Politics and Society* 31, 2 (2003) 325–55.

Smith, Steven Rathgeb and Michael Sosin. "The Varieties of Faith-Related Agencies." *Public Administration Review* 61, 6 (2001) 651–70.

Stewart, Francis. "Relaxing The Shackles: The Invisible Pendulum." Paper presented at Development Studies Association Conference 2008, "Development's Invisible Hands". Church House, Westminster, London: 8 November 2008.

Stiglitz, Joseph E. "Forward to 'The Great Transformation," in *The Great Transformation—The Political and Economic Origins of our Time*, by Karl Polanyi, vii–xvii. Boston, MA: Beacon Press, 2001.

Stringer, Martin, "Introduction: Theorizing Faith," in *Theorizing Faith: The Insider/Outsider Problem in the Study of Ritual*, edited by Elisabeth Arweck et al., 182–86. Birmingham: University of Birmingham Press, 2002.

Swartz, D., "Secularization, Religion, and Isomorphism: A Study of Large Nonprofit Hospital Trustees," in *Sacred Companies: Organizational Aspects of Religion and Religious Aspects of Organizations*, edited by N. J. Demerath III et al., 323–30. New York and Oxford: Oxford University Press, 1998.

Swinton, John and Harriet Mowat. *Practical Theology and Qualitative Research*. London: SCM Press, 2006.

Taylor-Ide, Daniel and Carl E. Taylor. *Just and Lasting Change: When Communities Own Their Futures*. Baltimore: Johns Hopkins University Press in association with Future Generations, 2002.

Tearfund. *Transforming Lives: Church-Based Responses to HIV*. London: Tearfund, 2007.

The Capacity Project. "Working with Faith-Based Organizations to Strengthen Human Resources for Health," in *Capacity Project Knowledge Sharing*, May 2007. 1–2.

The Salvation Army. *Orders and Regulations for Field Officers*. London: The Salvation Army, 1891.

———. "The International Social Council, 1921." London: The Salvation Army, International Headquarters, 1921.

———. *Handbook of Salvation Army Doctrine*. St. Albans: International Headquarters, Campfield Press, 1923.

———. *The Salvation Army Year Book 1990*. London: SP&S, 1989.

———. *Salvation Story—Salvationist Handbook of Doctrine*. London: The Salvation Army, 1998.

———. *The Salvation Army Year Book 2000*. London: SP&S, 1999.

———. *Mission in Community*. London: The Salvation Army International Headquarters, 2005.
———. *Salvationist Ecclesiological Statement—The Salvation Army's Place in the Body of Christ*. London: Salvation Books, 2008.
———. *The Salvation Army Year Book 2010*. London: Salvation Books, 2009.
———. *Building Deeper Relationships Using Faith-Based Facilitation*. London: The Salvation Army International Headquarters, 2010.
———. *The Salvation Army Handbook Of Doctrine*. London: The Salvation Army International Headquarters, 2010.
Thiemann, Ronald F. "Lutheran Social Ministry In Transition: What's Faith Got To Do With It?," in *Taking Faith Seriously*, edited by Mary Jo Bane et al., 177–209. Cambridge, Mass.: Harvard University Press, 2005.
Thomas, Stephen, et al. "The MESH Approach: Strengthening Public Health Systems For The MDGs." *Health Policy* 83, 2–3 (2007) 180–85.
Thompson, Judith. *SCM Studyguide to Theological Reflection*. London: SCM Press, 2008.
UNAIDS. *Partnership with Faith Based Organizations—UNAIDS Strategic Framework*. Geneva, UNAIDS, 2009.
United Nations Development Programme. "The Global Strategy for Women's and Children's Health" in *Human Development Report*. Online: http://www.un.org/sg/globalstrategy.shtml.
Van Der Geest, Sjaak, et al. "User Fees and Drugs: What did the Health Reforms in Zambia Achieve?" *Health Policy Plan*. 15, 1 (2000) 59–65.
Varman, Rohit and Ram Manohar Vikas. "Rising Markets and Failing Health: An Inquiry into Subaltern Health Care Consumption under Neoliberalism." *Journal of Macromarketing* 27, 2 (2007) 162–72.
Walker, Pamela. *Pulling The Devil's Kingdom Down - The Salvation Army in Victorian Britain*. Berkley and Los Angeles, CA: University of California Press, 2001.
Wallace, Anthony. *Religion: An Anthropological View*. New York: Random House, 1966.
Webster, Robert. "Health of Soul and Health of Body," in *Inward and Outward Health: John Wesley's Holistic Concept of Medical Science, the Environment and Holy Living*, edited by Deborah Madden, 213-232. London: Epworth, 2008.
Wells, Samuel. *Transforming Fate into Destiny: The Theological Ethics of Stanley Hauerwas*. Carlisle: Paternoster Press, 1998.
Wesley, John. *The Works of John Wesley*. Grand Rapids, 1872.
———. *The Works of John Wesley*. Nashville: Abingdon Press, 1986.
Williams, Harry. *Every Army Needs An Ambulance Corps*. London: Salvation Books, The Salvation Army IHQ, 2009.
Winston, Diane. *Red-Hot And Righteous—The Urban Religion of The Salvation Army*. Cambridge, MA: Harvard University Press, 1999.
Wittberg, Patricia. *From Piety To Professionalism—And Back? Transformations of Organized Religious Virtuosity*. Oxford: Lexington Books, 2006.
Woodall, Ann. *What Price The Poor? William Booth, Karl Marx And The London Residuum*. Aldershot: Ashgate, 2005.
World Health Organization. "Declaration Of Alma-Ata International Conference On Primary Health Care, Alma-Ata, USSR, September 6–12, 1978." Online: http://www.who.int/hpr/NPH/docs/declaration_almaata.pdf.

———. *Building From Common Foundations: The World Health Organization and Faith-Based Organizations in Primary Healthcare*. Geneva, World Health Organization, 2008.

———. *The World Health Report 2008: Primary Health Care Now More Than Ever*. Geneva, World Health Organization, 2008.

Xu, Ke, et al. "Understanding The Impact of Eliminating User Fees: Utilization and Catastrophic Health Expenditures in Uganda." *Social Science and Medicine* 62, 4 (2006) 866–76.

Zizioulas, John D. "Human Capacity and Human Incapacity: A Theological Exploration of Personhood." *Scottish Journal of Theology* 28, 5 (1975) 401–47.

———. *Being as Communion: Studies in Personhood and the Church*. Reprint of 1997. New York: St Vladimir's Seminary Press, 1985.

———. "On Being a Person: Towards an Ontology of Personhood," in *Persons, Divine and Human—King's College Essays in Theological Anthropology*, edited by Christoph Schwobel et al. Edinburgh: T. & T. Clark, 1991.

Index

African Christianity
    secularisation of, 5–6
African context
    HIV/AIDS flood of donor dollars, 73–74
African governments
    view of churches' involvement in health services, 42
African Health Strategy (2007-2015), 42
African Religious Health Assets Programme (ARHAP), 7, 8, 69, 73
aid
    to make individuals better off, 47–48
aid interventions
    Australian focus on process of outcomes, 44–45
AIDS *see* HIV/AIDS
All the World, 106
Alma-Ata declaration, 16–17
    call for emphasis on primary health care, 53
anthropology
    of the body and soul, 128, 136, 157
    Booth's conception of, 101
    SA's theological, in a state of flux, 103–4
    Wesley's theological and relational, 90–91, 93–94, 102
ARHAP *see* African Religious Health Assets Programme

Asia, South and East
    commodification of health care, 49
Atherton, John, 50–51
atonement
    Booth's insistence on centrality of, 115
Augustine, 141
    Church inhabiting an alternate space, 19
    the Church in the *saeculum*, 137–38, 139
    conception of the two cities, 137–39
    and the importance of worship, 144
    reflections on health, 126, 130
AUSAID *see* Australian Agency for International Development
Australia
    focus on process of aid interventions outcomes, 44–45
    SA's corporate success in, 6
Australian Agency for International Development (AUSAID)
    engaging with churches in PNG, 63
"autonomous rational individual"
    juxtaposed against the concept of "healthy persons", 23, 51, 157, 165
    and less defined concept of community, 55
    myth of the, 49–51, 73, 86
    as pinnacle of human existence, 135
    result of the Fall of humanity, 132

Index

secularizing concept of persons, 165, 171
serving market and state solutions, 25, 133

Babylon and Jerusalem
  Augustine's conception of two cities, 137-39
Bane, Mary Jo, 75
Barth, Karl, 145
Bebbington, D. W., 110
Beccattini, Giacomo, 51
Begbie, Harold, 111
Benedict, Saint, 148
beneficiaries of funding
  risk of loss of ownership, 171
Bevans, Stephen, 9
Bible
  key to understanding of "healthy persons", 125
bio-medical establishment
  many skills they are unable/unwilling to offer, 150
bio-medical model of health care
  arguments against, 149-50, 160
  continually pushing towards expansion, 150-51
  dominance of, in Ghana, 162
  dominating health services, 149
  proving too costly, 84
  reliance on, 79
Blair, Tony, 168, 169
Block, Fred, 31
body and soul
  Booth prioritizing soul, 101-3
  Booth's and Wesley's conceptions, 102
  prioritizing body, 132
  SA rejection of body-soul dualism, 104, 157
  Wesley's concept of symbiotic relationship, 90-91, 102
Bolivia
  SA's integrated health program in Cochabamba, 160-61
Bond, Linda, xiii-xiv, 158-59

Booth, Bramwell
  message to SA Social Work Council, 113-14
  proposal to open up hospitals in India, 99
Booth, Catherine, 94, 102-3
Booth, Charles, 95
Booth, William
  address at SA International Social Council, 111-12
  eschatological *telos*, 106-8
  grand plan, 97-101
  motivations, 94
  problem analysis, 95-97
  on role of faith in transformation, 97
  seven "essentials to success", 96-97
  theology of atonement, sanctification and incarnation, 115
Bretherton, Luke, 11, 15, 24, 26, 32, 66, 68, 78, 127, 136-37, 148, 152, 167
Brock, Brian, 156

care
  integrated continuum of, 60
care of sick people
  tensions in functioning of market-state, 31
carers
  market demands for, in west, 33
Caspary, Almut, 130
Catholic health care
  in USA, 81-2, 82n
Cavanaugh, William, 19, 24
Chikankata Health Services
  complex relationships and resource demands, 42-43
  trendsetter for SA, 39, 39n
children
  death rates, 12, 13
Christ
  true direction of creation's teleology re-established in, 136, 137
Christian
  as member of the body of Christ, 131

Christian Church
  SA situated firmly within wider, 117–19
Christian eschatology
  and secular, 4–5
Christian minority settings
  institutional-based health ministry in, 4, 146
Christian mission hospitals *see* hospitals
Christian social institutions
  loss of links with denominations, 81
Christian theology *see* theology
Christians
  marginalized minority in India, 36
  in Papua New Guinea, 61–62
Church
  the institution of the, 141–46
  provider of social services in PNG, 63
  role in congregation-based health care, 83–86
church growth
  in developing countries, 79
church hospitals *see* hospitals
Church and the world
  defining difference between, 142
church-state partnerships *see* partnerships
Churches Health Association of Zambia (CHAZ)
  Memorandum of Understanding with MOH, 41-42, 41n
Churchill, Sir Winston, 155
city of God, the new Jerusalem
  and the earthly city of Babylon, 137
civilized culture of conflict
  conception of relations, 58–61
clinic-hospitals
  in the community, 83, 85, 86, 87, 164
  encouraging state to partner with church in, 151
  envisioning a faithful role for, 140
  in Ghana, 161–62
  seeking the characteristics of hospitality, 150
  value of, in hostile communities, 4, 146
Cochabamba
  SA's integrated health program in, 160–61
Collier, Paul, 45–47
commercialization of health
  impacting health of the poorest, 15, 18
commodification
  community vulnerable to, 55
commodification of health care
  FBOs as a "countermovement", 32
  sick person as a burden, 32
  in South and East Asia, 49
"common ground"
  becoming a priority for the SA, 71
  interrelated roles and practices as basis for, 75–77
  legitimate concerns when making partnership, 75
  the search for, 71–77
  seeking, in African context, 73–74
  sustained by FBOs living out beliefs, 76
commonalities
  between FBO typologies, 70
communitarianism
  variations in approach, 54
community
  emphasis shift from family to, 53
  health institution as a resource, 83
  notions of, 53–55
  term to be handled with care, 122–23
  western donors preferring to invest in, 78
Community Health Workers (CHWs)
  training schools for, in PNG, 62
community-based initiatives
  preferred to congregation-based, 85–86
community-based primary health care
  offering space for meaningful dialogue, 150
  see also primary health care

community-based programs
    for children with disabilities in Ghana, 162
    self-help groups in India, 38
community-centric responses, 52–55, 77
community/hospital-based care
    identifying the issues, 3–4
congregation-based health ministry, 83–86
    positive reviews and potential tensions, 86
    risks in developing, 165
    supporting Kenyans affected by HIV/AIDS, 176–77
    trend for FBOs to promote community-based over, 165
congregations
    brought into contact with suffering, 147–48
    and FBOs, tensions in relationships, 42–43
    as public benefit organizations, 84
    relevance of, x-xi
"Constantinianism"
    priorities of Church and of worldly powers, 141–42
corporate culture
    challenges confronting FBOs, 6–7
Coutts, John, 105

Dale, Gareth, 30, 31
de Gruchy, Steve, 85
death rates
    of children, 12, 13
denominations
    loss of links with Christian social institutions, 81
Descartes, René, 128
development aid
    identification of Christianity with, 5–6
dignity and rights framework
    for establishing "common ground", 72–73
disease burdens
    affecting developing world, 13–14
disease-specific funding
    problems associated with, 14, 18
    see also funding
doctors
    pressures on Indian, 36–37
doctrine
    Handbook of Salvation Army Doctrine, 104, 107n
domestication
    of the Church, 20–21
donor funds
    and donor priorities, 171
donors
    influence of external, 43
    influence on policy, 44–45
    see also funding
dual mission
    of SA, but not a dualist soteriology, 105–6
dualism
    dangers of body-soul concept of, 128
    of personhood, SA's, 103–4, 105, 157, 159
    priority of soul over body dismissed, 120
    in soteriology, Booth resisting, 112
    Wesley's, 90

Easterly, William, 47
ecclesial character
    for SA, articulated by Needham, 117–19
ecclesiological ambiguity
    created by William Booth, 117
ecclesiology
    of SA, 107n
    SA ceasing to observe sacraments, 107, 167
    sacraments in traditional worship, 166–67
    six key points for a Salvationist, 118
economic behavior
    questioning traditional assumption of, 50

economic globalization
    affecting rural and urban communities, 33
economically developing countries
    proposal to exclude from MDGs, 45–47
economy of wellbeing, 51
engagement
    civilized "culture of conflict" as means of, 58–61
England
    Booth on problems of the poorest in, 95–97
eschatological imperialism
    SA's purpose of "saving the world", 107
eschatological postponement
    rejecting a theology of, 120
eschatological *telos*
    Booth's, 106–8
    of "healthy persons", 139
    importance of, for Christian Church, 119
    revised, for SA health ministry, 139
eschatology
    tensions between Christian and secular, 4–5
eternal health
    Wesley's focus, 91
Etzioni, Amitai, 53–54, 55
evangelistic efforts
    abandonment of foreign missionary, 80–81
evangelizing and social services
    the SA's dual mission, 104–6
Evans, Abigail Rian, 80, 84
Evers, Adalbert, 52, 56–61, 74, 87, 110

facilitation approach
    with tools infused with faith-based insights, 172
faith
    modern medicine needing people of, 134–35
    reluctance of FBOs to articulate, 6–7
    resurgence in matters of, 67
    role of, in character transformation, 97
    variations of, within FBOs, 69
    see also other faiths; people of faith
faith dimension
    in framing of initiatives, 5
faith-affiliated organizations
    Sider and Unruh's typology, 71
Faith-Based Facilitation (FBF), 173
    FBF process in five stages, 174
    tools to support FBF process, 174–75
faith-based health ministry
    addressing advice to withdraw treatment provision, 151
    concluding vision, 176
    counter-movement resisting market forces, 34
    envisioning a wider role, 150
    involving people of faith in the world's suffering, 148
    orientated towards "healthy persons", 136
    requiring greater emphasis on PHC, 164
faith-based institutions
    marginalizing influence of western libertarians, 55
faith-based movements
    rooted in congregations, xi
Faith-Based Organizations (FBOs)
    addressing advice to withdraw treatment provision, 151
    alert to forces shaping health landscape, 44
    analysis of market and state spheres of operation, 29–34
    called to engage in the *saeculum*, 145
    challenge to produce evidence of quality health outcomes, 176
    context of ministry, 56–61
    determining relations with state and market forces, 32
    and faithful hospitality, 149

forging "common ground" with secular liberal states, 75–76
health workers welcomed by people of all faiths, 146
identifying the issues, 1–2
increased government funding for in USA, 67–68
lacking resources for inter-disciplinary conversation, 7
landscape, 66–69
in a location of "tension dwelling", 151–52
marginalising effect of western libertarians, 55
move away from funding hospitals and clinics, 78, 80
need to re-envision responses to illness, 134–35
partnerships see partnerships
perceived as a "useful" asset, 15–16
preferring community-based initiatives, 85–86
recommended to couple with worshipping congregations, 165
reluctance to articulate faith, 6–7
search for an orientation for, 23
turn towards, supported by global health establishment, 16
typologies, 69–71
see also Third Sector
faith-based process
in transforming social relations, 170–74
faith-centered organizations
Sider and Unruh's typology, 70
faith-permeated organizations
Sider and Unruh's typology, 71
faithful hospitality see hospitality
faithful practice
SA in Bolivia and Ghana, 160–62
see also habits and practices
faithful presence
calling to, 138–39
faithful relationships
building in hostile communities, 146

faithfulness
recovery of, 154, 157
and transformed social relations, 168
the Fall
implications of, 130–36
Wesley's view of health in terms of, 90
families
Booth's concerns for, 99–100
family
focus for informal responses to health concerns, 53
FBF see Faith-Based Facilitation
FBOs see Faith-Based Organizations
Felleman, Laura R., 90
Fergusson, David, 142–43, 145
field reflections
from India and Zambia, 34–43
from Papua New Guinea and Netherlands, 61–66
field workers
resources for SA, 173
Foucault, Michel, 132
free markets
arguments against, 30–31
funding
for Chikankata Health Services, 39, 42–43
for congregation-based health ministry, 84
donor funds and priorities, 171
from western donors, 71–72
importance of *telos* of funding agencies, 165
increase of, for FBOs in USA, 67–68
influence of donors on recipient government policy, 44–45
preference for disease-specific, 14–15
Zambian attempts to address, 40–42
funding decline
for institutional health care, 82

Ghana

government funding for health services, 161–62
Gifford, Paul, 5
Glenn, Charles, 64–66, 80, 116
global economic downturn
    impact on MDGs, 45
global practical theology
    area for further work, 175–76
globalization *see* economic globalization
God
    being made in the image of, 127, 129
governance
    history of poor governance in PNG, 63
Gowans, John, 157–58
Green, Roger, 94, 106
Gunderson, Gary, ix-xii
Gunton, Colin, 128

habits and practices
    integration of, in SA health programs, 160–62
Handbook of Salvation Army Doctrine, 104, 107n
Hattersley, Roy, 105
Hauerwas, Stanley, 5, 24, 92, 93, 126, 131–35, 140–49, 151–52, 165–66
health
    the fallen state of, 130–32
    Wesley's understanding of, 90, 91–92
health care
    commodification of, in India, 36, 49
    FBO, countering against commodification, 32
health care institutions
    contributing to an integrated health system, 82
health expenditure
    growth in world's, 12–13
health inequalities
    between and within countries, 13
health institutions
    development, 79
    negative view of, 78

as a resource in the community, 83
    see also clinic-hospitals; hospitals
health insurance
    market-based option, 48–49
health issues of mutual concern
    requiring faith-based process to address, 170–74
health ministry
    clinic and hospital-based, 78–83
    congregation-based, 83–86
    institutional responses a challenge, 99
    integrated, socially embedded, 163–64
    reforming, 164
    SA theology of, 119–20
health of the poorest people
    introducing the issue, 12–18
health services
    African governments' view of FBOs, 42
health systems
    disruption of disease-specific funding, 14
    influencing shaping, 15
healthcare
    commodification in South and East Asia, 49
"healthy persons"
    concept of, 23–24
    confronted by illness and suffering, 132
    different from "autonomous rational individuals," 23, 51, 157
    as persons-in-relationship, 126–29, 136
    redeeming, 136–40
    shifting the focus to, x
    telos of, 24, 125, 136, 139, 154, 156, 157–60
    their humanity, location and uniqueness, 127
healthy relationships
    healthy people in, xi
Higgins, Edward, 113

Hindu nationalism
  rise of, in India, 67
HIV/AIDS
  congregation-based health ministry, 170–72
  flood of donor dollars, 73–74
HIV/AIDS funding
  concern over imbalances, 14
  FBOs impacted by donor dollars, 73–74
Holifield, E. Brooks, 102
holiness
  concerns over contemporary practice in SA, 122
  individualistic conception of, 167
  Wesley's emphasis on, 92
Holy Spirit
  over-dependence on the work of the, 167
  under-emphasis on the work of the, 144
  see also pneumatological eschatology
Homo oeconomicus, 49–50
hospital financing models
  in India, 37
hospital-based/community care
  identifying the issues, 3–4
"hospital-centrism"
  impacting health of the poorest, 14–15
  result of bio-medical approach, 149
hospitality
  achieving encounter, dialogue and understanding, 149
  Christian health ministry characterised by, 148–49
  as "eschatological social practice", 148–49
hospitals
  Christian mission, 78, 79–80
  costs of closure, 82
  experience in underdeveloped countries, 82
  Ghanaian pressure for development of, 162

the hospitable hospital, 146–49
mission, facing crisis, 83
placing limits on, 149–52
reorientation towards relational reflective process, 164
Salvation Army, in India, 35, 99
unsustainability of church-run, in India, 37
Zambian attempts to address resourcing, 40–42
see also clinic-hospitals
household
  importance of the, 53
Howard, T. Henry, 112
Howe, Brian, 6
Human Development Index, 61
human personhood see personhood
"humans"
  bearing the divine image, 129
  contrasting views of people, 49–50
Hunter, James Davison, 78, 138–39, 143–44
Huxley, Thomas
  criticisms of the Booths, 108

identity
  SA's multifaceted, 156
  significance of institutional isomorphism, 20–21
  through relationship, 126–27
illness
  as an opportunity for growth in faith, 132
  response when confronted by reality of, 131–32
In Darkest England and the Way Out
  Booth's grand plan, 97–101
  Booth's problem-analysis, 95–97
  the impact of, 110–14
  the legacy of, 115–16
in-between times see saeculum
inaccessible communities
  FBO's access to, 15, 18
incarnational theology
  and social conscience, 115
  social engagement of, 115, 116

Index

India
    Christian missionaries in, 34-5, 34n
    commodification of health care, 36, 49
    field reflections, 34–38
individual *see* "autonomous rational individual"
individuality
    concept of "healthy persons" enhancing, 135
Indonesia
    SA in Christian minority context, 4, 146
Industrial revolution, 25, 30, 90, 97
inequalities *see* health inequalities
"informal spheres"
    of human activity, 52
institutional capacity development
    SA's funding from AUSAID for, 63
institutional isomorphism
    FBO character affected through, 58, 72
    FBO vulnerability to, 168
    FBOs adapting to isomorphic pressures, 73
    not inevitable result of FBO partnerships, 72
    risks in church-state partnerships, 147
    through church sharing space with civil society, 20–21
institutional-based health ministry
    concerns about, 4
institutionalization
    of human care in Netherlands, 64
institutions
    Booth's proposals for, 98
    changing relationships, 81–82
    Christian social, 81
    expansion of church, in colonies, 79
    key role of, 78
    loss of credibility in twentieth century, 77
    problematizing, 120–21
    as servants of health and holiness, 140–52
instrumentalization
    of health services, 87, 165
insurance *see* health insurance
integrated continuum of care, 60
inter-faith partnerships
    for faith centered health care, 169–70
intermediary institutions
    value of, in serving hostile communities, 146
Islam
    Islamic NGOs, 67n
    SA programs well used by Muslims, 162
isolationist tendencies
    warning church against, 143
isomorphic impact
    of faith-based health ministries on congregations, 86
isomorphic pressure
    FBOs accepting secularized framework, 73
    linked to weakened institution/denomination ties, 81
isomorphism *see* institutional isomorphism

Jeavons, Thomas, 84
Jeremiah
    letter to the Israelites, 138, 139, 140
Jerusalem and Babylon
    Augustine's conception of two cities, 137–39

Kerela
    women migrating to meet demands for carers, 33
Kingdom of God
    established, if not fully manifest, 137
Kingdom of God on Earth
    and SA's role, 107
Kymlicka, Will, 54

Lawson, Kenneth, 108
liberal individualism, 50

libertarian suspicions
    marginalizing influence of, 55
listening skills
    key to practice of hospitality, 150
liturgy
    in search of faithful orientation, 24
    traditional worship practices, 165–66
location
    framing the question in terms of, 19–20
Lutheran World Federation
    Augusta Victoria Hospital, 170

MacIntyre, Alasdair, 22–24, 50, 74, 136
Maddox, Randy, 90, 104n
market
    case for conscious limits on freedom, 31–32
    faith in the, 32–33
    Polanyi's analysis of state and, 30–32
    ravages of, as Indian patients denied treatment, 36
market of approaches
    criticism of current, 48
market demands for carers
    loss of mothers from developing world, 33
market democracies
    Third Sector engaging with, 58
market forces
    fluctuations impacting on ordinary people, 31, 32
    Zambian reaction against, 41
market inducements
    for SA to train nurses in India, 34, 37–38
market liberalism, 30–31
market practices
    Booth's willingness to use, 98
market, state and community
    current realities of, 137
market-centric politics
    not a panacea for health of the poor, 49
market-centric responses, 47–49
market-related culture
    challenges confronting FBOs, 6–7
market-state
    care of sick people revealing tensions in, 31
    community vulnerable to commodification by, 55
    disembedding of social relations by, 59
    see also free markets
Mathewes, Charles, 137–38
MDGs *see* Millennium Development Goals
medical conditions
    benefitting from relational focus in health care, 164
medical missions
    rise of Protestant, 79
medical science
    Wesley's interest in, 91–92
medicine
    embedding in social relations, 163
    the fallen state of, 132–36
    individualization of modern, 134
    modern, in alliance with market-state, 133
medicine and health
    Wesley's understanding of, 90
methodological issues
    "insider" seeking insider-outsider perspective, 11–12
military terminology
    adopted by SA, 156
Millennium Development Goals (MDGs), 18
    not attainable without partnering, 68
    state-centric initiative, 45–46, 47
ministry
    health institutions in India as opportunity for, 38
mission
    SA's three-legged definition of integrated, 157–58
Mission in Community, 117
mission hospitals *see* hospitals

missionaries
  decline in number of western, in India, 35
  withdrawal of western protestant, 81
missionary doctors and nurses
  recent decline in numbers, 82
modernization
  linked with secularization, 66–67
Montiel, Hector Cuadra, 82–83
motive and practice
  among western Christians, 5
movement
  characteristic of faithfully present SA health ministry, 155–57
Mowat, Harriet, 10
Muslims
  Islamic NGOs, 67n
  SA programs well used by, 162
"mutual interest"
  established through multi-lateral endeavour, 150
  more realistic than "shared vision", 74
  multi-disciplinary quest for common ground, 75–77, 87
  partnerships based on, 151–52, 168–70

nation-state
  FBO partnering with, 152
national nuances
  conditioning rationales, 57
Needham, Philip, 117–24, 129, 159
"Neo-Anabaptist vision"
  indulging in unnecessary negativity, 143
Netherlands
  field reflections, 64–66
  "loss of the social middle", 64

Olivier, Jill, 7, 69
organizational character
  shaping, 21, 72
orientation
  need for Third Sector clarity regarding, 57–58
  or *telos*, a rich, dense concept, 22, 23–24
  Wesley's, 91
other faiths
  Christian minority settings, 4, 146
  congregation-based health ministry to, 171
  hospitality as means of encounter with, 149
Oxford Centre for Ecclesiology and Practical Theology (OXCEPT), 172–74

Palestinian people
  inter-faith dialogue on, 170
Papua New Guinea (PNG)
  field reflections, 61–64
Paris Declaration on Aid Effectiveness, 44
partnerships
  based on "mutual interest", 168–70
  choice of FBO partners, 72–77
  church/state, resistance to, 147
  congregations/clinic hospitals, 85
  interfaith, for faith-centered health care, 169–70
  legitimate concerns of FBOs, 75
  precondition for funding from western donors, 71–72
  with state and/or market providers, 151–52
  state/FBO, 68–69
  sustained by FBOs living out beliefs, 76
patient care
  charging systems for, in India, 37
patients
  Indian, inability to pay, 26, 49
  profitable and unprofitable, in India, 35–36
people of faith
  engagement with, in developing world, 67–69
  establishing common ground, 72

having access to inaccessible communities, 15
and health institutions, 77, 148
influence in development of Alma-Ata Declaration, 17
involvement at every link in care chain, 150
modern medicine needing, 134
time for reciprocity and relationships, 51
worship- and world-engagement, 144

perfection
concept of, 92–93

personhood
appreciation of the divine, 128
being made in the image of God, 126–27
Booth prioritizing the soul above the body, 101–3, 105
a claim to uniqueness in terms of hypostasis, 129
relational appreciation of, 120
SA official teaching on, 104, 105
theological concept of, 126
three-fold pattern of, 127

PHC *see* Primary Health Care
Plant, Stephen, 4–5, 107

pluralism
to be maintained by FBOs in USA, 68

pneumatological eschatology
call for greater attention to, 144
call for SA to prioritize process over form, 120–21
corrective to the managerialists, 156

PNG *see* Papua New Guinea

Polanyi, Karl
analysis of economic and social change, 25, 29–34, 56
contemporary reflections on, 32–34
and market-centric policies, 46, 47, 49
rejection of myth of *Homo oeconomicus*, 49–50

polis

the church as an alternative, 140, 153

poorest people
introducing issue of health, 17–18, 85

post-millennial eschatology
SA mission based on, 100, 106, 106n, 108, 117, 139

post-millennial theology
replaced by incarnational theology, 116

poverty
Booth on problems of the poorest, 95–97
in Papua New Guinea, 61

practical theological reflection
four-stage model, 10–11

practical theology
resources for people of faith to rely on, 176
seeking a more faithful *performance* of the gospel, 9

practices
integration of in SA health programs, 160–62
in work of practical theologian, 88

Praxis Model
offering an appropriate methodology, 9–10

"presence"
central to faith-based health ministry, 147

Primary Health Care (PHC)
church-run in PNG, 62, 63–64
faith-based health ministry requiring greater emphasis on, 164
focus of public health strategy, 16–17
local congregations well-placed to support, 85
under attack, 17

primary health initiatives
relational approach to health care, 150

process, faith-based

in transforming social relations, 170–74
professional practice
  development of resources for SA employees, 171–74
professionalization of care
  SA programs in USA, 66
proselytizing
  tensions over, 79
Protestant medical missions
  rise of, 79
Protestantism
  rise of an appreciation of the secular, 80

Railton, George Scott, 109
rationality tradition
  human person as body and soul, 128
RE *see* Religious Entity
redemption
  telos of redeeming "healthy persons", 136–40
relational approach to health care
  holistic appreciation of healthy persons, 149–50, 159
relational focus
  conditions benefitting from, in health care, 164
  strengthening of in SA work, 159–60
relationality
  divine origins of "healthy persons", 129
relationship with God
  distinguishing Christian communities, 167
relationships
  breakdown between Christian Church and society, 118–19
  as a "civilized culture of conflict", 58–61
  connecting people in an international, moral, 32
  denial of relational dimensions of personhood, 132

key to successes of ARHAP, 73–74
loss of institution/denomination links, 81
"manifold interrelations" of Third Sector, 56–57
tensions inhibiting ministry in Zambia, 42–43
using facilitation to build healthy, 172
see also faithful relationships
religion
  as ally of economics, 51
  extinction the evolutionary future of, 66–67
Religious Entity (RE)
  ARHAP term preferred to FBO, 69
"religious and non-religious elements"
  secularist demand that FBOs distinguish, 75–76
research
  the context, 3–8
  field visits and conferences, 8
  methodology, 9–12
  question of identity, location or orientation?, 18–25
Rudman, Stanley, 51, 128, 159

SA *see* Salvation Army
Sachs, Jeffrey, 45
sacraments
  SA ceasing to observe sacraments, 107, 167
  traditional worship practices, 166–67
saeculum
  Church in the, 137–38, 139
  SA living in the, 137, 139
  sustaining faithful presence in the, 146
Saith, A., 45
salvation
  Wesley's belief in developmental steps, 90
Salvation Army (SA)
  called to make a difference, xiii–xiv

ceasing to observe sacraments, 107, 167
Chikankata Health Services, Zambia, 39, 43
the Church, and a common *telos*, 117–19
critical of religious establishment, 100
defined, 2n
development of dual organizational structures, 103
development of social services, 110–14
diversity of initiatives, 155–56
the experience of, 3–8
fragmented theology in twentieth century, 115–16
hospitals, 34n, 34–35
International Doctrine Council, 117
International Social Council, 1911, 111–13
international vision statement, 15n
and Kingdom of God on Earth, 107
located within a typology, 70–71
mission, 104–6, 157–58
as a movement, 155–57
nurse education in India, 34, 37–38
relations with the state, 110
revised eschatological *telos* for health ministry, 139
social program, 59n
state pressures on, in Netherlands and USA, 65–66
theology and practice, 88–89
in the world, 108–10
Salvationist ecclesiology
Needham's six key points for, 118
sanctification
SA focus on, 103, 158–59
Wesley's account of, 92–93
Schön, Donald, 9
Scripture
key to understanding of "healthy persons", 125
sectarian tendencies
warning church against, 143

Sector Wide Approaches (SWAPs) initiative, 72
secular
Protestant rise in appreciation of the, 80
secular liberal state
and FBOs, quest for "common ground", 75–76
secular political consciousness
church percolating out into the, 145
secularist development thinking
increasing influence of, 4
secularization
of Dutch society, 64
as inevitable outcome of modernisation, 66–67
secularizing concept of persons
as "autonomous rational individuals", 165, 171
self-regulation of markets
misplaced faith in, 30–31
sick person
as a burden, 31
Sider, Ronald, 70, 71
single issue funding
problems associated with, 14, 18
Smith, Steven Rathgeb, 21, 72
social capital
of FBOs, 16
social engagement
Booth's commitment to, 105
of incarnational theology, 115, 116
social justice
emphasis on, 5
problematic as shared vision, 74
social relations
between different perspectives and faiths, 150
Booth alert to disembedding of, 96
Booth's plan for re-embedding of, 97–99
disembedding of, 25, 59, 60
embedding medicine in, 163
transfigured, priority for Christians, 167
social services

Booth's definition, 106
and evangelizing, the SA's dual mission, 104–6
SA institutionally based, 111–14
social significance
    Constantinian Church captured by illusions of, 142
social work
    SA becoming more institutionalized, 116
    SA international conference, 1911, 113–14
society
    breakdown in relations with Christian Church, 118–19
    "submerged tenth" of English, 95, 98–99
    tyrannized by agents of medicine, 133
Sosin, Michael, 21, 72
soteriology
    alternative, promised by modern medicine, 134
    Booth resisting dualism in, 111
    Wesley's, 90
soul
    Booth prioritizing above the body, 101–3
    SA rejection of body-soul dualism, 104, 157
"soul health"
    prioritised over body health, 131
space
    framing the question in terms of, 19–20
specialization
    of healthcare, 134
state
    pressures upon, affecting FBOs, 32–45
state domination
    of health care, in Zambia, 38–40, 42, 43
state funding
    for faith-based health ministry, 147
state intervention
    to repair damage by market forces, 31
state and market
    Polanyi's analysis, 30–32
state subsidies
    Dutch, influencing NGO policies, 64, 65
state-centric responses, 43–47
state-faith relations, 68–69
    turn to civil society in west, 15
state-led centralization
    in harmonization of donor procedures, 44–45
"submerged tenth"
    ignored by English society, 95, 98–99
suffering
    church learning from experience of, 147–48
    response when confronted by reality of, 131–32
supernatural healing
    embraced by Methodists, 91
Swan, Wendy, 106n
SWAPS *see* Sector Wide Approaches
Swinton, John, 10

Taking Faith Seriously, 75
Tearfund
    definition of the church, 7, 7n
teleology
    Wesley's, 91, 92, 94
telos
    "common ground" not formed by agreeing *telos*, 76, 87
    of healthy persons, 24, 125, 136, 139, 154, 156, 157–60
    mutual interest despite different, 74
    or orientation, 22, 24
    revised eschatological, for SA health ministry, 139
    SA conference report suggesting alternative *telos*, 113
    SA orientated by eschatological *telos*, 115–16

202   Index

sustained by a community, not individuals, 145–46
transcending the limited goods of practices, 22
tertiary care
  disproportionate focus on, 14–15
theological anthropology *see* anthropology
theological principles
  in congregation-based health ministry, 85, 165
theological reflection model
  based on Pastoral Care Cycle, 173
  resources accessible to SA social work employees, 172
theological resources
  side-lining of, 4
theology
  Booth's, of atonement, sanctification and incarnation, 115
  different models, 9
  in framing of initiatives, 5
  global, practical, 175–76
  and practice, 88
  telos of SA health ministry depending on its, 126
  Wesley's prioritized over medical interest, 91
  Wesley's two dimensional anthropology, 90–91, 102
  see also incarnational theology; post-millennial theology; practical theology
theology of health, healing and wholeness, 119–20
theology of mission
  SA's need for a, 117
Thiemann, Ronald, 75–76
Third Sector
  as hybrids, intermeshing, 59–60
  as part of mixed welfare system, 56–61
  role of constructive engagement, 59
  social and political role, 58–59
  in space between state, market and community, 60

tension field with "manifold interrelations", 56–57
see also Faith-Based Organizations
Third Sector strategies
  influences affecting, 57
Thompson, Judith, 173
trade unions
  Booth's reassurance to, 100
transfigured social relations
  priority for Christians, 167
treatment provision
  addressing advice to withdraw from, 151
Trevelyan, G.M., 101
Trinitarian mystery
  of persons-in-communion, 129
Trinitarian nature of God, 120, 129
  foundational to articulation of *telos*, 126
Trinity
  doctrine of the, 104, 128, 135–36, 157
trust
  need to rebuild, fitting well with FBO values, 16, 18
typologies of developing world FBOs, 69

UNDP *see* United Nations Development Programme
United Nations Development Programme (UNDP)
  Human Development Index, 61
United States Congress
  Charitable Choice legislation, 68
unity
  in organization, mission and message, 159
unity of purpose
  Bramwell Booth's conference paper, 113–14
  Higgins' message to SA, 113
Unruh, Heidi, 70, 71
unsustainability
  of most large faith-based hospitals, 78, 83

user fees
    market-based option for poorest people, 48

Walker, Pamela, 105, 111
Wallace, Anthony, 66–67
Washington Consensus, 33
    33n
Wells, Samuel, 165
Wesley, John
    on health and medicine, 89–94, 131
    prioritising importance of health ministry, 148
WHO *see* World Health Organisation
Williams, Dr Harry, 37
Winston, Diane, 109, 116
witness
    outside of church, validity to be tested, 145
Wittberg, Patricia, 81
women
    death rates, 13
Woodall, Ann, 105, 115, 116
World Health Organisation (WHO)
    on health inequalities between and within countries, 13
    on improvement in death rates of children, 12–13
    revised PHC approach, 17–18
    on trends undermining health program, 15
World Vision, 6n
world-engagement
    on the basis of encounter, 144–45
world-hating theology
    disagreement over, 143, 144
worship
    identifiable characteristics of Salvationist, 165–68
    key set of habits to sustain church, 142, 144

Zambia
    field reflections, 38–43
    political and economic transitions, 39
    state domination of health care sector, 38, 40–42, 43
Zizioulas, John, 126, 129

www.ingramcontent.com/pod-product-compliance
Lightning Source LLC
Chambersburg PA
CBHW051801230426
43670CB00012B/2377